Natural Beauty

PAMPER YOURSELF
WITH SALON SECRETS
at HOME

*L*AURA *D*U*P*RIEST

THREE RIVERS PRESS • NEW YORK

Published by Three Rivers Press, New York, New York.
Member of the Crown Publishing Group, a division of Random House, Inc.
www.randomhouse.com

THREE RIVERS PRESS and the Tugboat design are registered trademarks of Random House, Inc.

Originally published by Prima Publishing, Roseville, California, in 2002.

Random House, Inc., has designed this book to provide information in regard to the subject matter covered. It is sold with the understanding that the publisher and the author are not liable for the misconception or misuse of information provided. Every effort has been made to make this book as complete and as accurate as possible. The purpose of this book is to educate. The author and Random House, Inc., shall have neither liability nor responsibility to any person or entity with respect to any loss, damage, or injury caused or alleged to be caused directly or indirectly by the information contained in this book. The information presented herein is in no way intended as a substitute for medical counseling.

All products and organizations mentioned in this book are trademarks of their respective companies.

Interior design by Trina Stahl.
Interior illustrations by Laurie Baker-McNeile and Andrew Vallas.

Printed in the United States of America

Library of Congress Cataloging-in-Publication Data
DuPriest, Laura.
    Natural beauty : pamper yourself with salon secrets at home / Laura DuPriest.
      p.   cm.
    Includes index.
    1. Beauty, Personal. 2. Herbal cosmetics. 3. Skin-Care and hygiene I. Title.
RA778.D936   2002
646.7'042—dc21   2002072554

ISBN 0-7615-2099-6

10 9 8 7 6 5 4

First Edition

To my Mom and Dad,
Tony, Johnny, and Danny—
my inner circle

CONTENTS

ACKNOWLEDGMENTS

$\mathcal{W}$HEN I SAT down to write this book I had a 90-day deadline to meet. When my editor said, "Just write!" I shrugged my shoulders and began pounding away at the computer. It seemed like an easy thing to do, but what I later learned is that a book is seldom written without a dynamic team of people lending their talent and, most of all, support. I am wholeheartedly grateful to my large "A" team that stood behind this book and me. Their enthusiasm and overwhelming encouragement made it possible.

To Craig Harris, my team captain, who birthed the idea of bringing my natural recipes to television viewers, and produced our Emmy Nominated *Natural Beauty: Salon Secrets at Home* program at KVIE, Sacramento. You had the creative insight to see the potential for success. From the beginning stages of the program to the final pages of this book, you have been a constant, positive, and creative force. I will always be grateful for your leadership and for guiding me down the path of this beautiful, rewarding project.

Many thanks to the rest of the staff of KVIE, Sacramento, for the hand you gave in bringing about the *Natural Beauty* telecast and this book:

To Lori Glasgow, executive producer, for steering the show every step of the way. I am especially grateful for the on-air coaching and hot tea during the days of taping. You were a blessing.

To Pat Callahan, one of the original public television fundraisers whose spirit and enthusiasm helped me become a part of the public television on-air fundraising team. To Jan Tilmon for your insight in directing the show to public television nationwide, and for your kind introduction to Prima Publishing. To David Hosley, general manager of KVIE, thank you for supporting this project. To Leslie O'Brien, associate producer and the sweetest person I know. Thank you for all you did for me on the set and over the phone when I needed a writing coach. Your cheerleading and kind remarks pushed me to make it just a little better. You gave this first-time writer confidence and I will never forget your passion for making a project excellent.

And thanks to the rest of the hardworking folks at KVIE: Sheryl Gonzalez; Christine Watson; Roland Mills; Jan White; Lillian Nelson; my sidekick, Paula Long; Erik Pedersen; Eddie Collier; John Reed; Lou Galiano; Mark Johnson; Eileen Holleran; Jamie Judd; and Margaret Rodriquez. I knew, every step of the way, how hard you all labored to produce this book.

Thank you, Christi Collier, at American Public Television for your hand in bringing the *Natural Beauty* program to viewers across the country.

Thanks to Eric Swanson of River's Echo for your magnanimous Web management.

I'll never forget the day I met Jennifer Basye Sander, my acquisitions editor at Prima Publishing. I was shaking in my boots with excitement—and a little fear—when I was offered a contract. You helped me balance the thrills and the fears immediately. I am so grateful to you for steering me smoothly through the writing process and having so much patience with me. While I fretted about punctuation and style, you kept me focused on "just writing." I am so pleased to have had the opportunity to write a book under your guidance.

Of course I wish to thank Prima Publishing and all of their talented staff for their tremendous book production skills. To Michelle McCormack, thank you for making the final stages of this book so pleasurable. To Pat Henshaw and Jennifer Dougherty Hart, for your expertise in publicity; to Erica Hannickel, acquisitions assistant; to

Patti Waldygo for your copyediting talents; and to Andrew Vallas and Laurie Baker-McNeile for your wonderful illustrations.

To my parents, John and Joyce DuPriest, who taught me that one can accomplish anything. Besides providing a loving and encouraging upbringing, you helped out with many duties like answering phones during public television fundraising drives and assisting me with my boys. Most of all, I want to thank you both for passing along your good common sense, the basis of this book.

To my sister Linda DuPriest, a talented professional writer, for your gentle editing and cheerleading. Your "thumbs up" after reading my early chapters gave me the fuel to continue.

To my sister Nancy Owsley and her friend Mike Bowman, and to my brothers and their wives, Rob and Terri DuPriest and John and Renee DuPriest, for always helping me with my children.

To Dan Gray, my best friend and soul mate who was my mentor throughout the months of writing. Dan, you inspired me to write my favorite chapter, "Inner Beauty." You taught me how to say it "my way." I will never forget the hours of long distance calls that helped me forge ahead, one chapter at a time. You nudged me out of my writer's rut and helped research quotes. So much of this endeavor was made possible because of your constant coaching and encouragement.

My dear friend Tara Weyand deserves a super kiss and hug for all the hours of dedication she gave to me. Thank you for bringing me meals and for your artistry in developing the containers for the recipes. I love you.

To Kris Knutson-Kush who celebrated this book with me before it was finished. You held down the fort at my salon while I was at home writing. I will always be amazed at your competency and caring.

To my hardworking staff at the Laura DuPriest Salon and Day Spa in Sacramento, I share this book with you. You all helped make it happen. Many techniques in this book were researched and developed by you, my salon team. I applaud you.

To all of my salon clients over the past 21 years who taught me everything I know about the beauty business. Every single person who gave me the privilege to touch him or her, touched me.

To Michael Patrick Gallagher and Tara Barry of Riverdance, who gave me a peaceful place on the road to write many pages of this book. Your dedication and discipline was contagious.

To my friends at News 10, KXTV, Sacramento, for your professional support and for honing my "on-camera" skills: Russell Postel, Margaret Mohr, Jennifer Smith, Dan Elliot, Alicia Mallaby, Matt Elias, and Kevin Hale.

To Vi McNally of McNally Public Relations for endless hours of hard, but enjoyable, work. It's amazing to see how big the tree grows when you plant a tiny seed.

To David Schwartz at ABI in Sacramento, Janice Watkins, and Tony Walker for your generosity and computer support.

To Barbara and Wayne Carson, my most special friends—I couldn't have done it without you.

For your quiet dedication and friendship over the years, I wish to thank Maureen and Fred Forbes, Muriel Johnson, Gunter Stannius, Marcia and Gary Reimers, Ilan Frank, Mark Parreira, Kristine Harvey, Diana Penna, Commissioner Demetrious Boutris, Stan Van Vleck, Liisa Niemi, and Steve Novack. The next time I see you, we'll share high fives!

Lastly, but most importantly, I wish to thank and acknowledge my beautiful sons, Tony and Johnny, for your patience and understanding when I labored for hours at my laptop at the kitchen table. Not only did you tiptoe around the house, you did the laundry, cooked, cleaned, and helped create some of the recipes presented in this book. I am so proud of you both and how you pitched in for Mom's project.

INTRODUCTION

ONE DAY I visited the most expensive cosmetic counter in my hometown: La Prarie at I Magnin. At age 24, I had spotted a tiny crease beside my left eye when I smiled, and my panic drove me on a quest to find the best skin-care product money could buy.

At the counter, I listened while a "heavily powdered" woman explained how a cream formulated with "sheep placenta" would solve my wrinkle problem. Thank goodness the price of the precious cream exceeded my budget and sent me away empty-handed. As I left, my mind tried to digest the concept that was just outlined to me. It seemed a little absurd, so I read the company's brochure over and over, trying to make sense of it.

A few days later, I encountered a woman in her sixties with flawless, perfect-looking skin. I was so impressed, I asked her what she used to keep her skin looking so young. She replied, "You wouldn't believe me if I told you."

I said, "Try me."

Her answer was, "Crisco."

Twenty years later, after many hours of training, research, and experimentation, I began writing this book. Inspired by my doubt in the claims of a cosmetic company and an acquaintance's beauty secret, I would like to share my own acquired salon secrets for natural beauty.

· 1 ·

Natural Beauty

KNOWLEDGE IS THE KEY

"Knowledge is power." FRANCIS BACON

OST WOMEN I counsel use one word more than any other to describe how they want to look: *natural.* It crops up in almost every beauty consultation. Each year thousands of women sit in my salon chair, seeking advice on how to look naturally beautiful. My 20 years of experience have taught me that despite all the glamorous magazine ads that catch our eye, the stunning celebrities whom we admire, or the supermodels we try to imitate, women want to look gorgeous in a natural way. They want natural beauty.

So, how do you look natural and beautiful? Do you have to be blessed with good genes and a family history of smooth, glowing skin? Or can you achieve natural beauty? This book suggests wonderful new methods to help you look and feel better.

The way you look when you get out of bed could be considered fresh and untouched. Is that really the natural look you're going for? Wearing no makeup is natural, right? And a clean, soap-scrubbed face is natural. Or how about not even brushing your teeth—is that natural?

We all have different standards when it comes to the fine points of beautification. Even though we'd like to roll out of bed looking naturally beautiful, some of us feel more comfortable using enhancements to achieve beauty. In this book I offer you my experience, skills, and talent to help you create a natural, attractive look. The possibilities are endless! The most exciting thing about the world of beautification is that the field is so vast. The cosmetics industry is overflowing with as many opinions as it has products. I studied beauty for more than two decades and have created streamlined tips to make natural beauty an everyday part of your life. Once you try these, you'll be eager to share them with your family and friends.

Not by Chance

SKIN AND HAIR CARE is ever changing and full of artistic expression, fulfillment, and fun. When I see women get excited about looking good and becoming more beautiful, I'm inspired to create new beauty routines for them. The first thing I do before making suggestions is establish what their standards are. Listening to my clients is very important. When I learn what they're seeking, I can help them reach their goals. Then we assess how much enhancement they desire or are prepared for. My job as a beauty expert is to figure out how to improve a client's looks and, more important, how to achieve the look every day. No one wants to spend two hours in the bathroom every morning getting ready to go out the door. People who spend that much time in front of the mirror usually look as if they do, right? Now, remember the magic word . . . *natural.* And imagine looking terrific, fabulous, alive, and beautiful—with the added bonus of seeming as if you were born that way.

How? I'll show you, step-by-step, how to capture the "natural beauty" look from head to toe. I'll help you bridge the gap that you imagine lies between you and the glamorous world of beautiful women. You, too, can turn heads and attract admirers.

I have a saying: "The more you know, the further you can go." Knowledge is the key; knowledge is power. Discovering all I could about "How to do it myself" is how I ended up in the salon business. I believe in *sharing* knowledge, not keeping it a secret. You may have discovered, as I did in my twenties, that many professionals in the salon business want to make a big mystery out of what they do. They want you to "need" them. The whole idea is to keep you attached to frequent salon visits. This is why you may feel that you can't style your hair or do your makeup as well as salon professionals can. But I say that you can. You just need to learn how. Who besides you should know how to best present yourself?

I'm a little different from some of the hairdressers and makeup artists you've worked with before. I love to tell my tricks and secrets! I get excited about teaching women and men how to look and feel better about themselves. I hope that you'll walk away from this book with a broad knowledge of the latest beauty secrets that will work for you and everyone you know. I'll also teach you to save time and money in the process. And I hope that you'll have a renewed interest in taking care of yourself not only on the outside, but on the inside as well.

GET INSPIRED!

❋

Look for natural beauty role models within your circle of friends or family. They can be an inspiration for your new natural beauty routine. Keep a folder of magazine pages featuring celebrities you admire who are great examples of natural beauty. Some of my favorites are Jane Seymour, Katharine Hepburn, Jodi Foster, and Téa Leone. Even when they wear makeup, they never look as if they do.

Back to Nature

WHEN I REFER TO *natural beauty,* I emphasize two main points: First, we've already talked about looking beautiful in a natural way. The second part is achieving beauty with natural products. In recent years there has been a huge marketing trend in the promotion of natural products. It started in the salon and day spa industry with pioneers like Aveda. Even the cosmetics "giant" Estée Lauder came out with its "Origins" line, designed to romance the naturalist in the marketplace. At the same time fashion gurus were taking steps toward the natural trend, I stood in my kitchen, mixing natural skin-care recipes and rolling my eyes at the huge cosmetics conglomerates rushing to ride the "natural" wave after so many years of pure, unadulterated chemicals.

"How dare they?" I wondered, as I whipped up another honey oatmeal scrub. During those beginning days in my kitchen, when I experimented with my new skin-care line, I realized that women wanted to chase the dream of being beautiful. I decided that my quest was to bring knowledge to the vulnerable hearts of women—women who would spend almost any amount of money to look better. I knew back then what I know now: that natural ingredients can make a difference in your skin, hair, and nails. More important, learning about natural products and their results can teach you the beauty basics. After reading this book, you'll be more informed about the entire beauty and cosmetics world. You will no longer be gullible, confused, or intimidated at the cosmetics counter, believing in and purchasing the next "miracle cure" for wrinkles. If I can teach you my salon secrets, you'll be better equipped to

EXPAND YOUR BEAUTY

❧

Take a quick survey of natural beauty remedies you already know about or currently use. As you read this book, add a new natural beauty tip to your routine each week.

navigate the "beauty maze" created by the media, the fashion industry, and the cosmetics counter.

Natural Beauty Debut

THIS BOOK CAME ABOUT because of a public television station production made in Sacramento, California, where I live. Craig Harris, a friend and producer, had heard about a local NBC news segment in which I introduced my homemade skin-care recipes. Many of these kitchen formulas were the beginning of the skin-care line I created for my first salon back in 1987. Craig believed that women would be greatly interested in homemade skin care, as an alternative to commercial cosmetics. Saving time and money were the focus of the show. I thought the show would be a fun new way to teach women about alternatives to commercial products that don't always live up to advertisers' promises. The audience response was overwhelming and gratifying.

On the first day of taping, as fragrant aromatherapy oils drifted through the air, female station employees clustered in our kitchen studio. They immediately embraced the ideas and wanted to learn more. In addition to their initial attraction to aromatherapy oils, the women were thrilled to discover the beauty benefits of common items found every day in their refrigerators and cupboards. The recipes I demonstrated were derived from skin-care science and common sense. The basics of skin care are easy to grasp when they are clearly explained. The women in the studio learned how skin functions and that taking care of their skin was easy. My goal was to dispel the myth that you had to spend a fortune on New Age products to look and feel good.

Since the first airing of the show, I've been amazed at the interest in this natural beauty concept. *The Natural Beauty: Salon Secrets at Home* show is currently airing on public television stations nationwide. Women are whipping up cleansers, acid treatments, and masks all over the country. My dream is that they'll be empowered to take care of themselves and look beautiful in the process. I'll continue teaching natural beauty principles to help women and men save money and avoid commercial cosmetics and creams that are often useless.

The Talent Within

REMEMBER, SALON PROFESSIONALS aren't miracle workers; they're just very experienced at manipulating hair, skin, and makeup. At one time salon employees were beginners, fresh out of school and with a lot to learn on the job. Your training is about to begin. While you go through the steps in this book, approach the principles as if you're going into the salon business. Forget your preconceptions about yourself, at least for a moment. Some people tend to be self-negative, doubting that they have the ability to improve or change. While you study these techniques, pretend that you'll use them on your mother, daughter, or best girlfriend. Digest the principles and hints first. Once you've accepted that my methods will work, apply them to yourself. Turn this natural beauty advice into a beautiful nature that you carry with yourself every day. You will glow from within. You'll notice a difference and so will others.

Science vs. Nature

THE BIGGEST QUESTION I get asked in interviews or via e-mail is whether I really mix up my honey and yogurt cleanser every night. I'll be the first to say that even though this method is important, effective, and fun, I usually use my homemade recipes mixed with commercial preparations. My usage is about half and half. When I can't conveniently mix ingredients in the kitchen, I rely on bottles of skin-care products on the bathroom shelf. Of course, my product of choice is my own skin-care line, which originated in my kitchen and contains many natural ingredients. My favorite natural recipe to use weekly is the sugar scrub. Mixing equal parts of vegetable oil and table sugar is the best, most effective exfoliator for the face. I believe in this formula. At age 45, I still get compliments on my complexion. My secret is a weekly dose of this natural scrub.

For You and Your Family

YOU MAY FIND, while reading this book, that members of your family will want to borrow it. Get everyone involved in chapter 6, "Facials from Your Fridge" and chaper 13, "Spa at Home." You can create a mini day spa right in your own home. Trade pedicures with your teenage daughter. You might actually talk your significant other into giving you a massage if you give one first. Many new discoveries of relaxation, pleasure, and fun are just around the corner for you and your family and friends.

One of the best viewer responses to the *Natural Beauty: Salon Secrets at Home* show was when we featured gift ideas. Children can learn to make their own bath salts for Mother's Day gifts. You can create a spa gift basket for around $10 with simple kitchen staples. The show even had a section devoted to baby items. And if you enjoy arts and craft projects, you'll love making your own spa creations with my recipes. You can give someone a gift of pampering and relaxation, a gift that really shows you care.

My Quest for Knowledge

IN ADDITION TO MY natural recipes and beauty secrets, I'll share with you my knowledge and experience from 20 years in the salon business and my former modeling career. I was a print, TV, and ramp model for nine years. At age 30, I knew I was crossing into the model's unemployment line, so I started a fashion production company. Over the next three years, I produced, choreographed, and directed over 60 fashion productions. A few chapters in this book are dedicated to secrets and tricks of the fashion and modeling world. I've had the rare experience of working on both sides of the stage and cameras. I have several licenses in the salon field: I'm a licensed manicurist and esthetician (which is a facialist and makeup artist), as well as a fully licensed cosmetologist (hairstylist). I'm also a massage therapist, spa therapist, and paramedical makeup artist. There is not a single service offered in my salon that I don't do. This is relatively rare in my field. Most people in the salon business nestle into one area and stay there for their entire career. I wanted to be knowledgeable in everything. As a salon owner, I wanted to personally train and guarantee the professional performance of all my staff. I found that the more specialties I mastered, the better I could understand all the different elements of beauty and self-improvement. If I could become a good makeup artist, I would understand hair coloring better because the two go hand-in-hand. If I could learn massage, I would be a better manicurist, because manicures incorporate many massage techniques. If I could become an excellent technical haircutter, I would be more precise at working with acrylic nails. I'm very proud that I can set the standard for all the services offered in my salon and day spa. I'm also able to zero in on a person's key features, from head to toe, and immediately spot the creative possibilities for someone who wants a makeover or a new style.

Wake-Up Call

I RECENTLY WENT THROUGH an entire makeover after ignoring myself for seven years. I made myself over from body to hair and makeup. I can personally tell you that change comes slowly, and for many of us, that's the only way we can handle it. When my youngest son was seven, I looked in the mirror and was shocked that I'd somehow gained over 50 pounds since his birth. I was the former model who'd planned to be back in my real clothes within six months. Instead, I bloomed slowly through his toddler years. In addition to the weight gain, I had let my hair drift into one of those easy-to-maintain poodle do's, I wore my glasses nearly every day and rarely got up early enough to put on makeup. I had evolved into everything I hated, a low-maintenance frump. Right about that time, I received an offer to appear regularly on a local TV show, mainly because I was considered an expert hairstylist and makeup artist. I was mortified at the thought of being on TV, which visually adds 10 pounds to a person. I was scared to death that my former modeling chums would see my failure. I turned down the show because I was embarrassed at my recent transformation from model to frump. I just didn't feel like a very good example of a beauty expert. I had lost myself along the way and set myself aside in the pursuit of children and career. I needed to regroup. My regrouping began with a careful analysis of what I would do, step-by-step, if a gal like me showed up at my salon to get a complete makeover. I thought of the advice I'd use to prepare her for a makeover debut. This hypothetical advice became my new plan. After a year and a half of reinventing myself, including diet, exercise, wardrobe changes, a new color scheme for my hair, a consistent skin-care routine, and makeup time in the morning, I now smile when I glance in the mirror. I finally gave a go-ahead to that TV show. By putting myself back together, I regained my confidence. The way we feel about ourselves on the outside has a huge effect on our insides—and vice versa.

Internal Medicine

SPEAKING OF OUR INNER selves—specifically, how we feel about ourselves—I encourage you to always think positively. Your outer beauty doesn't stand a chance if, inside, you are weighted down with doubt and negativity. The phrase "Beauty is only skin deep" is a cliché but, oh, so true. I have worked with some of the most glamorous and gorgeous women in the modeling field. Yet when they opened their mouths and negativity spilled out, my lasting impression was that they definitely lacked beauty. Your self-image should always reflect a happy and positive attitude. The world's most beautiful women, in my opinion, are those who are confident, poised, polite, and pleasant to be with.

Sharing Secrets

MY GOAL IN WRITING this book is to reveal the tricks of the trade directly to you. As you move from chapter to chapter, take what you need to create a natural, more beautiful you. You may begin to regard the salon, makeup counter, and modeling business differently. I promise that you'll learn something new and hope you'll have fun with your new beauty routine. Most of all, I hope you'll see yourself in a more positive light in comparison with others, and that you'll simply enjoy being naturally beautiful.

Please share this knowledge. Teach your friends and family the principles in this book, or, better yet, share a recipe with them. I believe that beauty is a way of life, not a competition. I want everyone to know what worked for me. I want these "secrets" to be beauty solutions, not a secret code only for salon professionals. I want to empower you to take charge of yourself and have fun doing it. Design your own look, and I'll help you achieve it.

Once you've learned the secrets and start digesting this new knowledge, it will make sense to include it in your life. Beauty is not something you have to achieve overnight. New habits, like a better skin-care routine or a new way of shopping, are difficult to change quickly. Let yourself be a work in progress. Throughout the book, I'll remind you to approach things this way. You may even want to read the entire book before you start to make changes. By simply reading these pages, you'll take the first step toward natural beauty and making time for yourself. Congratulations!

· 2 ·
The Model vs. the Mirror

*"She got her looks from her father.
He's a plastic surgeon."* GROUCHO MARX

THE BIGGEST PROBLEM I see when it comes to beauty is the high standard we set for ourselves! Most women, including myself, look to the image-makers in the fashion and beauty world, and then try to imitate what we see. I call this habit "The Model vs. the Mirror." Women devour glamour and fashion magazines, looking for beauty secrets and hopelessly comparing their own self-image to the sea of gorgeous faces in the supermodel world. We've all done it, right? I started out at 17, pouring over the pages of—what else?—*Seventeen* magazine, in search of anyone I could relate to. As I moved into my twenties, I graduated to *Mademoiselle, Glamour,* and then the big "doosey," *Vogue.* I studied the lipstick ads, surveyed the "how to" articles, and even tried to figure out from the editorials "who would ever wear those weird clothes?" As I moved from magazine to magazine, I thought I could never measure up to the beautiful girls who graced those fashion pages. I could never be beautiful. Beauty was way out there, beyond my grasp. I just wasn't born looking like that.

Comparing ourselves to supermodels in fashion magazines or beauty ads makes us feel that this level of glamour is unattainable. The beautiful models are high up on a pedestal, and we're down here in the real world. We couldn't possibly reach their heights of beauty.

Well, I say you can, or at least come very close. The key is to understand that what you see in those magazines or on the runways is a carefully orchestrated illusion. Most women don't realize that this illusion is created by a team of professionals and artists who are pretty darn good at their jobs. Behind the scenes of every fashion ad, editorial, TV commercial, or fashion show is a talented photographer, lighting specialist, makeup artist, hairstylist, wardrobe artist, and choreographer or art director. I know because I've been there, not only behind the scenes as a hairstylist and makeup artist, but as a professional model, fashion show choreographer, and producer. I've not only seen the creation of illusion with myself as a model, I've created the illusion with other models. I wish everyone could go backstage or in the studio before the transformations take place, to see the models when they walk in the door before the magic begins.

Models Aren't Goddesses, They're People

MODELS COME IN MANY shapes and sizes, just like you. The difference between you and them is simply that they were picked to be in an ad or a fashion show. The number one reason they are in the spotlight is because someone recognized that they had a particular physical attribute that would attract attention, drawing the public's eye to whatever the model will advertise. It's as simple as that. Now, I'll admit that many models have amazing physical attributes and are extraordinary in one way or another. Some people are just born lucky. Many models, however, are not gorgeous, but are rare in other outstanding ways. For instance, they may be exceptionally tall and lean, have a long and graceful neck, or have remarkable features like full lips and huge blue eyes. We've all seen high fashion models who are not particularly beautiful but who have an exotic or unusual look, just different enough from the rest of us to attract attention.

I have a good friend who is a plastic surgeon. One day during his haircut in my salon, I asked him about supermodels and their thin thighs. I wanted to know if they all had undergone liposuction. He chuckled. His explanation for women with no fat on their thighs was that they were "mutants" because they are so rare and unlike most women. His opinion, based on what he's seen in his practice, was that many had undergone liposuction. Others are extremely lucky. He said that if they had not yet had children, they might be lean enough to be fat-free in the thighs. After childbirth, women tend to pack fat around the thighs, which aids in lactation. His words made me feel a little more comfortable about my own thighs and my reality. We can all accept our self-image if we realize that we're closer to normal than the few lucky women with flawless bodies who walk around on the planet. I now think of those rare women as aliens to our planet; they are rare occurrences in nature, not the norm. They are "Einsteins" in the world of beauty, and we can't all be "Einsteins."

People have varying degrees of intelligence. By the time we are adults, most of us have a pretty good idea where we stand in the "brains" department. We seem to be pretty comfortable with our brainpower and intellectual selves or at least have accepted what we were born with. Our comfort level doesn't seem to sway even if we know that more intelligent minds than ours are out there. I personally don't get intimidated by watching *Jeopardy* anymore. I accept that others are more "brainy" than myself. So here's the question I want to pose to you: If we are able to accept the superintelligence of rare minds like Albert Einstein's, why are we so heavily influenced by "Beauty Einsteins"?

The answer is because we've trained ourselves over the years to be a highly visual society. Everything today is about visual stimulation.

Blame it on the media, if you want to, but the media only gives the public what it seems to demand. Newspapers and magazines wouldn't sell if people didn't buy them. TV ads wouldn't matter if we simply turned off our televisions. We—especially women—are the ones who demand a high beauty standard. We buy into it, spend money to achieve it, struggle to attain it, and then complain about having to live up to it. I'll show you how to understand and manage the "beauty pressure" in a more realistic, reasonable, and natural way.

THE ILLUSION

Let's go back to the illusion, or the magic of making the model that perfect image. This is what happens at a typical fashion shoot for a cosmetic ad. The model arrives at the photographer's studio in the morning, usually with no makeup on and clean hair, though it's probably still damp. The team of magicians begins to get her ready for the camera.

Makeup

The makeup artist will spend anywhere from 45 minutes to two hours detailing her face for the look the art director is going for. The advertisers in most fashion magazines retain some of New York's and L.A.'s top makeup artists, and I mean *artists*. The changes that develop during the makeup sessions would astound you. The point I'm trying to make is that any woman in the hands of these top makeup artists would look amazing when they're finished with her.

Lighting

One of the keys to the talent of makeup artists is their knowledge of the photographer's lighting set-up. Usually, photographers have a few favorite makeup artists whom they work with. It's important that makeup artists understand how the photographer lights and shoots. They work in tandem to create the illusion. The way the photographer lights the model greatly determines what the makeup artist will use for cosmetics and how these will be applied. There's a saying in the modeling business—and I took it to heart when I was a model—"Be kind to your makeup artist and worship your photographer." Together, they can make or break you.

Hairstyling

Once the makeup is done, the hairstylist takes over. The first thing I want you to understand is that hair can be manipulated and faked in a million ways for photo shoots, fashion shows, and even TV commercials. Wigs and extensions are often used, as well as many expensive hairpieces that are time-consuming to put on. Natural hair can be teased, rolled, ironed, textured, and arranged in many ways—of course, by the hairstylist. Models don't do their own hair. They have a lot of help. Remember this when you look longingly at an editorial or an ad, and you desire that perfect hair. The model did not get out of bed that way. Try not to compare yourself to the model. I recall a fashion shoot I did in San Francisco in the 1980s when hair was big and full. I have thin, fine hair, but got hired for the job anyway. The hairstylist rolled my hair, teased the heck out it, and then pulled an age-old trick out of his bag. He parted my hair in the back of my head and pinned the hair toward the front, securing it right behind the ears. By transferring all of my hair from the back to the sides, he made my hair look tremendously thick and full. From the front, I looked great. If I turned around, you could see a bizarre array of silver clippies and a "Pippi Longstocking" part down the middle. This worked for the camera, but would be hard to pull off walking down the street.

As a hairstylist on photo shoots, I've worked with models who had very dry and damaged hair from all the styling that had been done to it. To get the look and, of course, the "shot," I'll do whatever it takes to get the hair looking perfect. The miracle products for hair these days make it pretty easy. Spray glosses, leave-in conditioners, waxes, pomades, and super-holding hairsprays will allow a hairstylist to literally mold and shape the hair to do just about anything. Without these tools, the model's hair probably looks like yours, straight out of bed in the morning.

WALK THE WALK

When walking down the street, pretend you are on the runway in Milan or Paris. Feel like a model. Stand up straight and walk as if you're wearing the most expensive garment in the world. Chin up and strut!

Wardrobe

The final step to creating the illusion is the wardrobe. I've had the good fortune to wear some of the most expensive and beautiful garments in the world. From Donna Karan to Armani, I walked the ramp clad in the very best. When you put on a $6,000 silk gown, it instantly changes how you feel about yourself. Maybe it's the quality of the fabric, or just the power behind how much the gown costs. Whatever the case, wearing designer fashions makes you feel like a million bucks. When you feel good, you look good. Attitude is everything, in my opinion, when it comes to looking great. I'll speak more about this later in this book.

The Crew

Finally, let's talk about the photographer, the art director, and the rest of the crew. I never worked on a photo session where I didn't temporarily fall in love with somebody. When you're a model and surrounded by a crew working hard to make you look your best, you're suddenly seduced into believing that you are a queen, at least for that day in the studio. Everybody on the job coos and fusses over you. The photographer oozes endearing phrases and cheerleads you along into the illusion you were hired to embody. At the moment the camera and strobes go off, you know that you're the most gorgeous woman on the planet. The encouragement and approval from the crew were the only reasons I ever bought into the idea that I might just possess a little beauty. I had to be talked into it. I wish that all the women in the world could land just one high-powered photo session and be treated like supermodels. It's a true confidence-builder.

The Mirror, Your Friend

SINCE WE CAN'T PROJECT ourselves into the modeling world every day, we need to remember that beauty and glamour can be created. This should empower you. When you look in the mirror, focus on what you see as the starting point. Imagine what you would like to improve. Start believing that with a little effort, you can easily accomplish these changes.

Later in this book I'll talk about inner beauty and how external beauty begins from the inside out. The way we feel about ourselves greatly affects how we appear to others. For many women, looking in the mirror immediately brings up negative thoughts. The mirror becomes our enemy when we try to maintain a positive outlook. I've witnessed this so many times at my salon. Even the prettiest of women look in the mirror and cringe with disappointment over what they see. Sometimes my cheerleading can snap them out of their negativity, but many women have gotten into the habit of being overly critical with themselves. Ironically, being

SEE THE LIGHT!

Did you know that you can see the lighting that was used to make a model look beautiful? Look at the reflection of the lights in the model's eyes. It may help to remind you that the photographer's lighting and talent helped to create the model's glamorous image. She's a human being just like you. Trade places with her and imagine how great you would look!

self-critical is extremely unattractive. Why point out to others that something's wrong? Why beat up on yourself?

As a beauty adviser, I've developed an exercise to encourage a better relationship between you and the person in the mirror. I call it my "Number 3" rule, and I practice it daily. Here's how it goes: When you get up in the morning or before you leave the house, look at yourself in the mirror and point out three great physical attributes that you possess. Also do this each time you're aware of a negative thought about your outer self. For instance, you get up, get ready for work, glance in the mirror, and see that your hair is not at its best. Instead of focusing on the hair disappointment, find three things in the mirror that please you. You may say to yourself, "I like my blue eyes, my skin is looking especially clear and glowing today, and I feel good about staying on my exercise plan." Now that you've reset your thinking, you might enjoy restyling your hair. The Number 3 rule, when practiced daily, will become a habit of creating goodwill. It's similar to strategies used in the workplace. When I train employees, they're more open to constructive criticism if I first compliment them on several things that they have mastered well. Progress is difficult in a negative environment. I encourage you to incorporate this positive approach in your daily routine, especially when you get ready in the morning. Slowly but surely, the mirror will not be a source of negative thinking. It will become a friend and a source of pride and confidence.

TAKE A SHOT!

❖

Have a photo session with a professional fashion photographer in your city or hometown. You may be surprised at how you are transformed through the talented eye of a great photographer.

Observe and Admire

As I LEARNED MORE about changes I could make to enhance my features, I began to look at models and celebrities differently. Instead of being jealous or feeling inferior, I became an admirer. Now I strive to be a quiet observer and look for the beauty in other people. We can learn a lot from the way beautiful women present themselves. Appreciating beautiful women is similar to appreciating art. Before I studied art, from the classic masterpieces to modern works, I didn't "get it." I didn't have the knowledge to understand and appreciate paintings and sculpture. After a few art courses, I was empowered with enough of the basics to understand art. This understanding led me to a heightened sense of appreciation. My admiration for art in all forms continues to grow.

Look at beautiful women around you and learn from them. Let them be a guide and inspiration as you learn more about your own beauty. Include yourself in the group of women whom you admire.

· 3 ·

Landing the Look

"There's only one corner of the universe you can be certain of improving, and that's your own self." ALDOUS HUXLEY

IN ADDITION TO my salon experience, I became very involved in the fashion industry. My introduction to the fashion world came as a bit of a shock, when I was asked to participate in a local TV commercial. I had never worn a lot of makeup and didn't consider myself model material. I knew nothing about looking glamorous. I caught on when I was thrown into the fire. I learned by watching and imitating. I followed—or at least, limped along—in the footsteps of the other models.

When I had my fill of life as a model, I drifted to the other side of the curtain, producing my own fashion shows. My skills at imitation stretched into the roles of choreographer and fashion coordinator. I quickly learned by trial and error how to put together a show full of outfits and ensembles. I'm grateful for the mentors who helped me shape my fashion instincts. I tapped into the artistic skills of many designers, store-owners, department-store heads, and fashion consultants. Now these skills can guide you.

You're the Architect!

IN CHAPTER 1 YOU learned how important it is to take control of your own "exterior design." You are your own architect. You get to choose your own style and create your new look. I see the opportunity to redesign myself in the same way that I might redesign the interior of my home. I usually find a plan or style that I like and try to imitate it. Let's say that you decide to remodel your living room. Chances are, you'll gather up some home-improvement books or magazines to get ideas, a little inspiration, or the most up-to-date trends in colors and furnishings. Most of us remodel our homes because we like a fresh new look. Changing a room around is fun and exciting; it makes our lives more interesting. The same can be true for our bodies and physical appearance.

When people come to my salon for makeover advice, I try to learn a little about their lifestyle. I begin by asking about the style of their home, what type of furniture and accessories they like, and even when they last bought something new for their home. This last bit of information gives me some insight into what their limits of change are. Not everyone is comfortable with change, but many people spend a lot of time and energy keeping up with the latest in furnishings and home décor, yet spend little or no time on themselves. It's rare to see anyone with orange shag carpet from the 1970s in their living room, but I still see men and women with 1970s hairstyles. Your appearance gives the world an impression about you. If you enjoy presenting a beautiful home, you'll find it equally rewarding to present others with a beautiful you.

To begin to "remodel" yourself, you need ideas, inspiration, and a plan. You know that you need an update, but you're not sure what your personal design should look like. We already discussed the danger of trying to imitate the unrealistic supermodel image. This chapter will help you "land the look" that you can feel comfortable with and can achieve on a daily basis. In it, I include many ideas from creating fashion shows, as well as tricks I learned from numerous artists and staffers at boutiques, retail stores, and department store chains. I'll teach you a new way to research your look in fashion magazines and how to shop more efficiently.

My Makeover Story: Frump-Itis

BEFORE TAKING YOU DOWN your new design path, I'd like to tell you the details of my personal makeover that I mentioned in chapter 1. It began the day I realized I'd become part of a new trend I'd noticed. It's not my desire to be overly critical or judgmental, just to point out a condition that I think is choking the beauty out of women. I myself caught this malady at age 35 and had it until recently, when I found the "cure." I call it *frump-itis*.

"FRUMP-ITIS"

I first heard the word in high school. If a teacher looked like an old school marm, she was labeled a *frump* or she "looked *frumpy*." To me, the term meant "old-fashioned" or "out of date." In the salon I hear this word tossed around a lot, mostly by clients describing what they *don't* want to look like. I decided to do a little survey one day and asked several clients what that word meant to them. The response was varied, but generally, most men and women said the same thing. According to the clients surveyed, *frumpy* means "out of date, somewhat unkempt, behind the times, antique, and uninteresting." When I asked if men could be frumpy as well as women, the answer was usually yes. When I asked if one could look frumpy even at age 19, the answer was also yes. Everyone agreed that frumpy could describe men or women, was not a respecter of youth, and was always negative.

In the late 1990s, I, too, suffered from "frump-itis." It wasn't something that happened overnight, but slowly evolved after my kids were born. I suppose I had ignored the changes that occurred as the busy months rolled by. It was easy to set aside my fears that I was gaining weight. As I began to trade up my clothing for larger sizes I stopped looking in the mirror, even when I went shopping. I shopped for things that felt comfortable. Most of the time, I simply didn't care how I looked in the garments. My first indication that I had changed was when I developed an old roll of film and discovered that the woman in the photos—me—was someone I didn't recognize. That same day I went to the mirror and noticed that I looked a lot different from my trim, fit, glamorous model days. In just a few years, I'd eased into a frumpy hairstyle; stopped wearing makeup; wore glasses instead of contact lenses almost exclusively; and chose clothes that hid my soft, overweight body. I had turned into a frump, for sure.

Looking back, I can see how it happened. When I had my babies, I became overwhelmed with the daily tasks of life and reasoned that taking care of myself should take a back seat to bottles, diapers, day-care schedules, and my job. The funny thing is that my job was making other people look good. Even though I worked, day after day, in front of a mirror at my salon, I never looked at myself in the mirror; I just focused on the clients' reflections. As the kids got older, I thought it would be easier to take time for myself, but the diapers were replaced with their school, homework, and class projects. The habit of tuning myself out became my way of life.

One day I was in a discount store, trying on some jeans. It seemed that all the jeans I'd bought that year were shrinking rapidly. As I tried to squeeze into a 14 (my modeling size was a 4 or 6), I looked hard into the mirror and let my brain catch up to the evolution of the last eight years. I actually did not recognize myself. I didn't even look like a female. I was clad in a baggy T-shirt, with a baseball cap covering the permed, quick, and easy hairstyle that I thought was cute. The hairstyle was not cute, and I was not beautiful.

I didn't buy those size 14 jeans. As I headed for the front door, disgusted at the weight I'd gained, I checked out other women in the aisles. I saw a sea of women who looked just like me. Everywhere, I saw women in baggy jeans or sweats, large T-shirts, athletic shoes, and a lot of baseball caps. Not one single woman really stood out, not a single female had a great look. I'm not talking about just clothing. I didn't see anyone who looked like anything except straight out of bed or straight off the sofa. *Where had all the beautiful women gone?*

Later that day, I relayed my sad jeans story to my mom. I asked her if I looked like a size 14. She said yes. I was stunned. Even my sweet mom saw it. I had gained a lot of weight and I was a frump. During the 30-mile drive home from Mom's, I had a long talk with myself. I needed to change. I knew I had to go back in time and try to figure out where I'd gotten out of the habit of taking care of myself.

I reflected back to the year I'd left my modeling career. I was 30 years old, 120 pounds at 5'8". I was not only trim, I was toned and fit and always felt as if I could turn heads in public. I wore a current hairstyle and always a little makeup, mostly blush, mascara, and lipstick. I felt good about myself and never agonized at the reflection in the mirror.

I now believe that I started to look frumpy as I gained weight. In looking at family photos, I realized that I'd started to lose control of my weight just after my second child was born. I never restored my pre-pregnancy body, and I just seemed to look worse as the years rolled by. In my young modeling years, I spotted a few women over 40, looking old, tired, and frumpy. I swore to myself back then that I'd never let myself get like that. I'd never lose my figure or give up on putting myself together. Well, it turns out I did exactly what I'd declared I would never do. And I did it without being conscious of it. I woke up two years ago at the age of 43 and had my "mirror crisis." I owned one of the top salons in Sacramento, the capital of California, but I certainly didn't look the part. What kind of advertisement was I for my own business? It bothered me . . . a lot. I needed to regroup, to go back and find the real me.

In the process of this reassessment, I looked around at women I knew, both in my salon and around town. That's when I figured out that I wasn't alone in the neglect zone. Women in general have drifted away from fixing themselves up. Have you noticed it, too? Aside from the Annual Academy Awards show or a televised beauty pageant, when do you see women striving to look terrific and glamorous? The world has turned a little too casual and comfortable perhaps, or maybe we've just bridged the gap between men and women too much. We don't seem to make the time to be beautiful.

Now you may be saying, "So what? Why should we women have to fix up? Men don't have to." Well, no one *has* to. We could all get out of bed, throw on any old clothes, and slump off to work. I believe, however, that most women still want to be noticed and admired. I witness it every day in the salon. I'm solicited daily by women to help them look better. Women want beauty answers. I'm convinced that beauty is still a goal for even the busiest of women.

I want you to go back in time, 10 or 20 years ago, when women truly looked different. Back then, when I was modeling, I used to love to go to the nicer stores like Saks, Joseph Magnin's, or Liberty House and see all the beautiful women decked out for a shopping trip. I remember saying that I wanted to look just like them when I launched my career and earned some good money. Those women seemed to have a great deal of pride in the way they looked. They were always well dressed, wearing makeup, and sporting a nice hairstyle. Even though they were only out shopping, they looked great.

Many of the women whom I admired back then didn't work and raise children. I think that today's working women—especially working moms—have too much on their plates. It's not that we want to ignore ourselves, it's just that we've shifted our energy away from ourselves to balance a career, husband, kids, soccer practice, PTA meetings, and so on. When on earth is there time to get fixed up every day? But maybe time isn't the only factor. Maybe pride has something to do with it as well.

Not taking time for ourselves is just part of the equation. Time is only one issue contributing to "frump-itis." Other factors are habits and lack of knowledge and trends. Women walk around on the planet imitating each other. We like to travel in packs, shop together, lunch together, work out together, and, eventually, we dress alike. I believe that women themselves are responsible for the spread of "frump-itis." If our girlfriends are okay with casual frumpiness, we'll tend to accept the look for ourselves. Women encourage each other to be frumpy and so it is perpetuated.

THE UNISEX TREND

Over a decade ago, Calvin Klein, one of my favorite designers, came out with his CK line of clothing and cologne. The concept of this line was unisex, jeans that fit and were styled for both guys and girls. His cologne was supposed to appeal to both sexes. I thought it was a great concept, sort of a unification of men and women, a more simple approach to fashion. I think the uni-look worked well for 19 year olds. Then an interesting trend started to develop, as more designers jumped on the unisex bandwagon. Women became a little too comfortable dressing and fragrancing themselves like men. I believe that the blending of both sexes in the fashion world is one of the chief causes of "frump-itis."

WOMEN STARTED DRESSING AND LOOKING LIKE MEN

The next time you're out at the mall, the grocery store, or the hardware store, especially on the weekend, take a visual survey of the women you see between ages 20 and 60. Chances are, you'll see a lot of sweats, jeans, big T-shirts, athletic shoes, Flintstone-like sandals, and warm-up suits. I jokingly say that today's women look like a hockey team on the weekends. (I used to be the captain of a team, so I should know.) Many women are at least 30 pounds overweight. It's hard to tell men from women if you don't take into account the hairstyles.

The day I drove home from the dreadful jeans incident in a Target store, I stopped at the market to buy some Slim Fast and a whole pile of fashion magazines. I wanted to go through the magazines and figure out what year it was and what I was supposed to look like. I needed to discover where I went down the wrong fashion path. I had to redefine how I wanted "me" to look. I needed inspiration, creativity, and, most of all . . . hope. I didn't want to look like a guy. I didn't want to look as if I had given up. As I rounded the corner to my driveway, I had a revelation: If I didn't want to look like a guy, I had to get rid of my guys' clothing.

Get the Guy Out of Your Closet

This might go a little against the grain, but I guarantee that you'll begin to get it as you search for your new look. Go through your closets and drawers and take out all of your clothes that were styled for a man. Hold up each piece of clothing and evaluate it. *If a man would feel comfortable wearing it, get rid of it.* Take a hard look at the mountain of weekend and casual clothes you've purchased over the years that you selected because they were comfortable or you thought they were fashionable. Once I did this, I realized how much I had de-feminized myself. I was shocked that almost all the casual clothes I owned could have been worn by my brothers. I couldn't believe that I had outfitted myself almost entirely in masculine garments.

Now, you may reject this closet cleansing and think that you need comfortable casual clothes. You may say that it shouldn't matter what you wear on the weekend or around your house. I challenge you that if you take this step, you'll rediscover a sense of pride in looking like a woman.

When I did this exercise, I ended up with three garbage bags full of various T-shirts, baggy jeans, men's shorts, boxers, and sweats, which I carted off to the Goodwill store. I decided that day to never again buy one piece of clothing that a man would feel comfortable wearing. Now my number one fashion guide is to buy only clothes that better display my feminine side. *If a guy would wear it, I won't buy it!*

I hope that as you read this, you're taking a mental inventory of what's in your closet and drawers. Start with what you're wearing now. Would your husband or boyfriend wear it if it were their size? I've told my new fashion rule to many male friends, and they all agree that it's a good rule. Many of them say how great it is to see a woman dress like a woman. Men like us to look like girls. They like to see a difference.

Once I got rid of my guy clothes, I had a new sense of pride. All of a sudden, I wanted to take a few extra minutes styling my hair. I started wearing perfume again, and I actually enjoyed the time I spent putting on cosmetics. I had a sense of worth that I hadn't experienced in a long time. I enjoyed being a female and taking a moment to make myself presentable. All of a sudden, doing my hair and makeup wasn't a chore, it was a joy . . . fun. Imagine that.

After raiding and depleting my closet, I realized that I needed to get some basic items of clothing. I couldn't really afford a whole new wardrobe, and, don't forget, I was at least 60 pounds overweight. I had topped out at 194 pounds, which was a lot for my 5′8″ frame. I decided to start with one pair of slacks and a couple of tops. I made a mental point of planning to look for garments with a feminine touch.

Architectural Plan: Before You Go Shopping

HERE'S WHERE YOUR PLAN comes in. I always encourage women to get a mental picture of what they want to look like before they go shopping. Most of us just grab a girlfriend and head to the mall, the goal being female bonding and spending. The danger here is that you usually end up with a hodge-podge of clothes that may not be the best choices for you. We often get caught up in the event of shopping, instead of buying what we really want or need.

You need to establish your "look." Your image or personal style should be well defined before you go shopping. Models and their agents know that this secret is very important to a model's marketability. You can design any look you want. Having a clear picture of what image you desire for yourself is the most important step to take before you go to the mall. Imagine that you're hosting a big dinner party for honored guests. You would certainly plan the menu and prepare a shopping list ahead of time before going to the grocery store. The same principle applies to your image plan. Make it a big event and plan accordingly.

Map Out Your Plan with Magazines

When I taught modeling classes to beginners, I showed girls how to read a fashion magazine. I still believe that magazines are the best tool for guidance and inspiration. Magazines are varied and geared toward different lifestyles and demographics. You'll know which magazine is best for you at a glance. I always recommend buying two magazines that appeal to you.

I use magazines for fashion, hairstyle, and makeup help. I rarely read the articles. I find most of them trite and repetitive and generally just don't have time to read them. If you cast aside the articles, break down the magazine into three resources:

1. Advertising
2. Editorials
3. Buyers' guides

Advertising

Fashion ads are great resources for educating yourself on trends and current styles. The creators of ads are the best in the business. The individuals behind any advertisement are the trendsetters and artists of the fashion and cosmetics worlds. I learned many makeup techniques just from studying cosmetics ads. The difficult thing is deciphering the message in extreme ads so that you can relate them to yourself. Some ads are way out there, so be careful.

In looking at an ad, try to pick out one idea from it. In a cosmetics ad, for instance, the message may be "gold highlights on the brow bone" or "dark red lips are in." In a shoe ad, the message may be "chunky heels." The ad may feature a ridiculous-looking model in a freaky hairstyle, which may not appeal to you, but you can relate to the "chunky heel" shoes. The elements that stand out and speak to you are the ones you'll want to remember when you go shopping.

Editorials

Editorials are usually composed of several pages of pictorials, with a little bit of commentary from the fashion editor. I really like editorials for two reasons. I like to see the new models who are selected and featured, and I like to see what trend is being forced upon us. Don't get me wrong; I enjoy seeing trends and the push toward change. I think that the ever-changing fashion world is refreshing and fun, but

I recommend that you take any fashion editorial with a grain of salt. All I want you to do after you skim the editorials is try to grasp one or two new fashion ideas. Never imitate the models on the pages exactly. Fully imitating the models in an editorial may cause you to appear overdone or too trendy. Some of the choices in editorials are outrageous and very overpriced. Just try to get the essence of the new fashion season. Look for the following key points:

1. Length of hemlines in skirts and dresses
2. Cut of pants: bellbottoms, slimmed
3. Color statement: what colors are in for the season
4. Solids or prints and patterns
5. Shoe silhouette: slim or chunky heels, round toes or pointed
6. Accessories: splashes of color, metallic, or classic
7. Fabrics: textured and heavy, or smooth and flowing

By training yourself to scan the editorials and grabbing the key points that the designers present, you'll have a better idea which designs are current and fresh. Staying current will give you confidence in your personal presentation. Choosing garments that fit the current look will make you feel up-to-date. Trying to incorporate these new ideas in your wardrobe will make you feel better about yourself and your self-image.

Buyers' Guides

Most fashion magazines have a section in the back to help consumers locate the clothing featured in the editorials. I used to bypass these guides, but I've learned that they can save me a lot of time when shopping. Take the time to look through the buyers' guide for the prices of featured garments. Find out before you go shopping if the clothing you admired is affordable for you. The guides will also tell you where to find the garments. Many times, they include phone numbers and directions on how to order by phone or on the Internet.

BUILDING YOUR WARDROBE

Start your new wardrobe with just a few basics. This is particularly important if you're planning a weight-loss program. You may be preparing for a body makeover and should not invest a lot of money on clothing purchases that may be too big in a few months.

I find that most women buy too much clothing anyway. Women tend to want a lot of different outfits, but don't necessarily choose clothing of quality. Well-dressed men, on the other hand, often have fewer pieces of clothing in their drawers and closets, but have better-quality clothing. Think about how a businessman dresses. He may have only one or two suits, but adds different-colored shirts and ties for varied looks. The price of a suit is an investment, but it's justified because a good suit will usually last several years. I have learned a lot from the way men shop. Now when I shop for a season, I'll purchase one really great suit or outfit, rather than several. I'll then buy a few coordinating tops and accessories to go with that one great outfit. I've learned that rotating my outfits more often suits me just fine. Women really don't need the variety they think they do. When you're shopping, go for quality, not quantity.

Your look should be well-thought-out before you go to the mall. To get a plan in motion, flip through a fashion magazine and mark or tear the pages of looks that appeal to you. Assemble them in a folder. You may have several pages because you like the pants on one page but the blazer on another page. You get the idea.

Now, repeat the procedure with a second magazine. Put the pages in your folder. This will be your "look book." Your look book will be the fashion plan that you'll take to the mall. From these pages, you'll

DON'T FALL

Shop for great-looking shoes, but make sure you can walk comfortably in them. Nothing will kill your look faster than poor posture or a limping gait.

begin to develop a definite style. Your style may develop very quickly. If so, it will be relatively easy for you to shop. Some women don't find this process easy or comfortable. If you go through magazine after magazine without pulling out a single page, chances are you're reluctant to see change. You may be unable to relate to the newer styles. Don't be alarmed or feel left out of the fashion loop. We all have our D-day; mine was that day in the Target store when I discovered my "frump-itis." As I poured over fashion magazines to find out where I went wrong, I became extremely discouraged. I felt so out of touch looking at those fashion editorials. I couldn't relate to anything, probably because it had been such a long time since I had really focused on glamour.

If you feel out of it and uncomfortable when you do the magazine scanning assignment, definitely don't go shopping. Give it another try in a week or two. Look around you every day and pick out some well-dressed women close to your own age. Take a moment to really notice what they're wearing. You probably just need to make yourself more fashion-sensitive. We all tend to desensitize ourselves when we get busy or involved in school, family, or jobs. Being fashion-savvy takes a little training, much like art or interior design training. You can teach yourself a little bit at a time simply by making yourself aware of the fashion around you. As you notice what others are wearing (which can influence you both positively and negatively), you'll begin to develop a good eye for fashion.

GET OUT THERE

If you feel out of touch with current fashion trends, find out if any stores are having fashion shows in your area each season. Most fashion shows are free and are a big help in tuning up your awareness.

OTHER GREAT INFLUENCES FOR YOUR LOOK

If you really feel out of the loop in designing a look for yourself, try some other resources.

1. TV shows
2. Movie characters
3. News or talk show hosts
4. Soap opera characters
5. Celebrities

Pick someone on television or in a movie whom you can relate to. I did this once after seeing a Meg Ryan movie, and had my look designed for a whole year. After watching the movie several times for its romantic value, I noticed how great her character looked and marched right out to buy an outfit like one she wore in the movie. One reason I push women and men in this direction is because it allows us to take advantage of some great fashion experts. Movie and television wardrobe experts are fabulous at defining the look of the characters they design for. It's all about communicating the look of the character. Most of the time the result is very specific. I enjoy the fact that Hollywood's top fashion designers and experts are out there showing us great designs. We can tap into that talent; it just takes a little observation.

I also recommend picking out the best-dressed news personalities in your area. Pick people who are close to your age and really focus on the way they present themselves. I work with a lot of media on-air personalities. The trend in news media has become more and more fashion-oriented, especially for women. Women news anchors are expected to be trendsetters, particularly on the national level, where there's fierce competition to be beautiful, as well as an intelligent communicator. Many of the women in network news could rival supermodels. Look to these women for updated ideas on wardrobes, as well as on hairstyles and makeup.

Women who don't work often remark that they feel out of touch with fashion because they are home and not among the workforce. I counter that with the reminder that daytime television is a parade of fashion. Focus on the talk show hosts and celebrity guest stars on their shows. If soap operas are your cup of tea, you can use them to stay up on the latest trends. Soap opera stars are usually on the hip side of fashion. I never get to watch daytime TV, but I try to glance at soap opera tabloid magazines at the grocery store. Many times, a client at my salon will specifically ask for a hairstyle worn by a soap opera star. I need to keep up with who's who and what they look like. I have found that men and women on soaps are not only gorgeous but also outfitted superbly.

Finally, you may choose to follow the personal lives of favorite celebrities—not in a movie or TV role, but in the way they attire themselves in real life. My personal favorites are Meg Ryan, Michelle Pfeiffer, and Charlize Theron. They each have a great sense of classic fashion, are never trashy, and are always individual. Whenever I catch them in a celebrity magazine, I always make a mental note of what they're wearing and, of course, their hairstyles. Their makeup is never overdone, very natural. You may already have a celebrity whom you admire or can relate to. Incorporate this person's image and style of dressing into your own plan.

DON'T BE SHY

When you spot a woman in a great-looking outfit, stop and ask her where she got it. She'll be happy to tell you and your asking her will get a smile. It's a win for both of you.

Off to the Mall

AS I MENTIONED EARLIER, have a list of the items you're shopping for before going to the mall. That's step one. Step two is really important: Go to the mall alone. I know that we women like to go in groups, or at least with a buddy, to shop. It has evolved into a social occasion. My recommendation for a solo adventure is so that you can focus on your own mission. You'll have more success without the influence of a girlfriend's opinion. Chances are, a buddy will keep you in the rut you've been in. You'll serve yourself better without a friend's input.

Know what your budget is before you step into a store. Your limit on spending will be a determining factor in which store you choose. Most fashion malls have a variety of stores with several price ranges.

Don't spend beyond your means. Feeling good about your purchases will make for a better shopping experience.

Take your look book into the store with you. Ask for help at the counter before you even look around. Explain to sales clerks exactly what look you're trying to put together and then let them help you with that look. Sales clerks are there to help you, so get out of the habit of saying, "I'm just looking." The clerks know their inventory and can save you a lot of time.

I've often walked right up to a sales counter, shown the clerk an outfit from a magazine photo, and said, "I am looking for something like this and I can spend $150. What can you show me in this price range?" You'd be surprised how ambitiously they'll put together a look for you. Don't be afraid to ask for help.

Help from Displays

Here's a great secret I learned when I produced fashion shows. I was often hired to put together a 45-minute fashion show, with as many as 20 models to outfit in more than 150 ensembles. That's a lot of fashion coordination, and it used to exhaust me. The goal was to go into a department store or boutique and in a very short time grab the essence of what was current and what to show on stage. Usually, I stood in the middle of the store and gazed up at the walls and central store displays. If I looked carefully, I could see that the entire fashion show was expertly laid out. Every store employs artists, fashion experts, and display personnel to "dress" the store. The really neat thing is that the store completely changes almost weekly. The displays are loaded with terrific ideas and are near duplicates of the fashion editorial pages from many magazines. All

Do It Right

Make a point to visit a large department store and meet the personal shopper. Ask her to help you define a new style for yourself. Even if you don't make a purchase, her feedback may be valuable in planning your future wardrobe.

you have to do is stop, look, and study for a moment. The high-impact garments are usually right up in the front windows of any store. Take your cue from these great displays. If a store is in your price range, go with the exact outfit that's on the mannequin. Each outfit will be complete and very tastefully done. It's almost like a "paint by number" lesson in fashion. The displays are usually placed right next to the rack of clothing being featured. Just waltz up to the rack and select your size. Voila! Instant "look!" Before I picked up on this little secret, I would sift through rack after rack of garments, not ever finding what I wanted. The problem was not having a clear idea of what I was trying to put together. Now I love displays.

Your Hairstyle

MORE THAN ANYTHING ELSE, your hair says the most about you. You could wear a great outfit and still look like a frump if you sport a frumpy hairstyle. On the other hand, you could wear jeans and a T-shirt and be instantly noticed if you have a great hairstyle. I'll go over your hairstyle in detail later in chapter 10, "Mastering Your Own Hair." You probably already have a feeling about your hair right now and know whether your style needs to be updated. Hairstyles change rapidly, but changing with the latest trends isn't always easy because we all have different hair types. Use hair and fashion magazines to become familiar with what's out there on the street. Take a closer look at how your hair looks now and what kind of style you'd like it to be.

Makeup

UNLESS YOU OVERDO IT, makeup always helps create a great look. As we women get busy with work and raising kids, the first thing we neglect is putting on makeup. I still encourage women to apply makeup in a way that looks as if they don't wear any. This is an area where I use the phrase "natural beauty." If we can really see the makeup, we're probably wearing too much. The trouble is, if we don't wear any at all, we women start gravitating to the masculine side of life. I'll outline for you a step-by-step approach to putting on makeup that will look natural and beautiful. I learned how to apply makeup from the best makeup artists in the business when I was a model. Makeup can be applied in less than 10 minutes, so none of us can rely on the excuse that we don't have time. It's as simple as knowing how. Makeup is a big part of your "look." It should become part of your personal style. Remember, it's one of the most important steps in setting us apart from men. I am personally grateful for the magic of makeup to help hide my flaws and bring out my better features. I make sure I set aside that 10 minutes to finish my "look." For more help with makeup, refer to chapter 8, "De-Mystifying Makeup."

Keep It Up

THE LAST THING I want to say about landing your "look" is to keep it up. Never give up on your personal style. It's a very important part of you. I have vowed never to sink back into my previous "unconscious" stage. From here forward, make a vow to never have a "bad year" when it comes to looking good. Buy a fashion and hair magazine for yourself monthly and take a little time to go through it. If you don't shop for yourself every month, at least shop quarterly. Always have in mind what you want to buy before going to the mall. Gather ideas for your next hair and makeup styles. Now that you're enlightened by the possibilities, it will be more gratifying and more enjoyable!

· 4 ·

Salon Snake Oil

"The pure and simple truth is rarely pure and never simple." OSCAR WILDE

F YOU'VE BEEN to a salon lately, you may have noticed that the entire front section is like a department store cosmetics counter. Many salons now host a myriad of bottles and products designed to entice you into spending money to chase the Fountain of Youth and eternal beauty. Gone are the days of a simple shelf of shampoo and hairspray. As you survey the items for sale, you may discover remedies for problems you didn't even know you had. Salons offer prescriptions for everything from dry skin to cellulite, from chemically treated hair to stressed-out nerves. If the salon you frequent is also a day spa, then you can count on even more products to lure you.

I am a "product junkie." Many of you probably are, too. I love to line the shelves of my bathroom with hair and skin-care products and fragrant shower and bath concoctions. I especially love aromatherapy products. It all has to do with taking good care of myself, and I enjoy it. The problem is deciding what works well and being assured that the retail items you purchase will do the job and are worth the price. I'm a big stickler on value when it comes to personal-care products, and I'm sure you are, too. If a product does what it says it will do, I'm enthusiastic about purchasing it. If the price seems reasonable, I'll definitely buy it.

After a hair service, you may find yourself at the counter with three or four items that your hairstylist recommended. Stylists are supposed to sell you products. That's part of their job. This chapter will give you guidelines on how to handle a stylist who encourages you to buy, buy, buy. I'll teach you to purchase only those items that you will truly use.

In the old days, during the Gold Rush and development of the frontier lands, an old wagon would pull into town where a proprietor would sell the townspeople liniments and remedies for everything from rheumatism to headaches. The phrase "Snake Oil" was coined for these remedies. The proprietor would hold up a bottle containing a mysterious fluid and begin a grand speech, making claims that the new tonic would cure all that ails you. The townspeople believed it because they wanted to. They spent any amount of money for the "Snake Oil," especially if the proprietor was charismatic and enthusiastic about his claims of magic. The believer who made the purchase often continued the myth, boasting to others how much better the tonic made him feel. From those early days of traveling "Snake Oil" salesmen to the claims made in today's salons, we the buyers are often too quick to believe whatever people tell us.

Intellectually, we may hesitate to believe everything we hear about a product, but sometimes we don't use our intelligence when purchasing. We use our emotions, and that's what most sellers hope for. This is particularly true when buying cosmetics and personal-care items that supposedly make us look or feel better. We have a powerful need to hunt for solutions to maintain our appearance. The cosmetics and personal-care industry banks on that need. Consumers spend billions of dollars every year to look better. Cosmetics and personal care is one of the fastest-growing industries all over the world.

When I first began in the salon industry 20 years ago, I felt gratified that in a salon, people could find the right information about skin, nail, and hair care. The products and services a consumer purchased in the salon were sold with honesty and integrity. We in the salon industry were professionals and purists. There was a big difference between products bought in a salon and those at overpriced cosmetics counters. Yet the need to compete with fancier brands sold at department store counters has created a new trend in salons. Many salon products on the market have drifted into the cosmetics counter mentality of unrealistic claims and high prices. As a consumer, you need to arm yourself with a little more knowledge to make wise purchases in a salon. Be on the lookout for "Snake Oil."

This chapter includes my impressions of salon products and services. Many services are extremely valuable to a consumer, yet others are sold much like "Snake Oil," promising amazing results but having little impact. I hope that you'll find this information to be valuable. As information solely based on my opinion, you may find it enlightening, or you may disagree with my findings.

Each state's governing board that covers cosmetology regulates most day spas and salons in the United States. In the last few years, regulations have become more stringent in an attempt to protect consumers from inexperienced hands. Licenses are granted to individuals after they receive an education and pass a certification test of some kind. The emphasis in testing is generally on client safety, in terms of cleanliness and knowledge about how services should be performed. You should feel fairly comfortable as a consumer that you will be handled in a safe manner. Most licensed salon professionals do their jobs very well.

Besides the hair or nail service, however, the job description of a salon professional usually includes being a salesman. Salons rely on retail sales to ensure profits. That's fine. As a consumer, you simply must be aware of the salon's desire to sell you products and must endeavor to find out whether what you're buying serves a real purpose.

As a salon owner, I train my staff to know what retail products we carry and how to use them. Of course, I want my salon to be profitable; it couldn't continue to exist without a profit. But my deeper reason for selling retail products to our customers is that I truly believe that salon products serve a need for the client. Can you imagine trying to cut and style someone's hair with just water? If I had only a towel and the shampoo bowl to use as tools, I could never design and style a customer's hair with the latest look in mind. As a stylist, I know the tools I need to create a great look. I use the right products to deliver the end result and, I hope, teach a client how to achieve the look at home. If this system of client education is done properly, then the recommended products become useful tools, not just a retail sale.

DO YOUR HOMEWORK

When considering a product to purchase, read the labels. You may not be able to understand all of the ingredients, but the instructions should give you a hint about the effectiveness of the product. Avoid products that boast unrealistic results.

So many times, we get home from the salon and look into our bag of goodies only to find that we are confused about what the bottles are for. It's not that we minded spending the money; we just forgot what to do with all the goop, right? If the product just sits on your shelf, and your hairstyle just sits there as well, the purchase was for naught. For this reason, arm yourself with a desire to know what the stylist recommends before you get to the counter and feel pressured to buy.

My first suggestion is never to buy a product that you do not see fully demonstrated. You should be in agreement with the stylist that it would be useful. If you don't understand the product's benefit or what to do with the product when you get home, then ask again. Unless this can be reasonably explained to you, don't buy it.

Let's take a tour of salon products, department by department, to better acquaint you with what's out there.

Hair Care

THE QUESTION I GET asked most often is: "What's the difference between a salon shampoo and the ones they sell in a grocery store?" Boy, is that ever a good question. In beauty college, they try to teach you that the best products are sold in salons and the crummy ones are sold in grocery stores. Well, that didn't sound very logical to me. I was raised on grocery store shampoo. My favorite one as a teenager was Herbal Essence because it smelled so great. My mom bought big sizes of grocery store shampoo because we had a large family and needed to economize. The shampoo worked fine, or at least I thought it did, as a teen.

Soap is soap, basically. Most any commercial shampoo will foam up and clean your hair, and if you're not extremely particular, you may choose to buy your shampoo anywhere at any price. For a lot of people, price is the deciding factor. For others, it may be the smell. Believe it or not, what drives most people to a particular brand is the packaging and the advertising. That's why cosmetics and hair-care companies spend so much money on advertising. It works. Besides being influenced by advertising, smell, and packaging, you should know what's in shampoo and other salon products and what they will do for you.

If you look at the label listing ingredients, the number-one substance in shampoo is water. That's right, most shampoos have water as the main ingredient. The good news is that you can stretch out how long shampoo will last by adding a little bit of water when the bottle is partially used. Shake it up and keep using. The second ingredient is usually either sodium laurel sulfate or ammonium laurel sulfate. Both of these will clean hair just fine, but alone, they tend to be a little harsh. The key to the difference in shampoos is what's blended with these two chemicals. This is where grocery store shampoo and salon shampoo differ. Without going over every possible ingredient, I'll simply tell you that the proof of whether or not a more expensive salon shampoo is worth it greatly depends on how particular you are. After many years as a hairstylist, I'm finally able to detect whether a client uses a salon shampoo. The hair feels different and many times will behave differently. Pantene and ThermaSilk are popular shampoos that are commonly purchased in a grocery store and work very well to leave the hair silky and shiny. My experience when working with clients who use one of these shampoos is that their hair won't respond well to a curling iron. The curls won't hold or last, due to the residue that the shampoo leaves behind. They work fine if you want silky hair, but I feel that they fail in the test for body and styling hold. At first I was amazed at this phenomenon; remember, I used to buy inexpensive shampoo. I can only tell you as a hairstylist that there is a definite difference from one brand to another.

The best way to see if you can tell a difference is to try different brands and discover what you like. An 8-ounce bottle of shampoo in a grocery store can range from $2.95 to $5.95, in a salon from $3.95 to $20.95. The higher-priced shampoos may offer essential oils, other botanicals, or safeguards like sunscreen. Try to find out from the salon professional why you should buy the shampoo she or he recommends. What special need will it serve? Then evaluate whether you think the price is warranted. If you buy it, decide whether it helped solve the problem it was suggested for and whether you noticed an improvement in the way your hair reacted. If the answers were all positive, then the shampoo is a good purchase. Finally, remember that in the salon and cosmetics world, the highest-priced product isn't necessarily the best one.

Hair conditioners are a little more complicated now. In the old days, you used to rinse your hair with lemon juice to restore the acid pH level to the hair after shampooing with harsh alkaline soaps. Next, creme rinses were created for detangling. Then, a whole new world of confusion opened up for consumers when conditioners were invented. At first, there was only one type of conditioner, the kind you applied in the shower and rinsed out every time you shampooed. Now we have other choices. There are leave-in conditioners that you apply after you get out of the shower and don't rinse out. There are deep conditioners for damaged hair that you apply once a week. Some hair doesn't need conditioners of any kind. The best recommendation I can give you for figuring out the myriad of conditioner products is to seek the advice of a hairstylist. Don't try to diagnose your hair in the grocery aisle. When stylists make a recommendation, ask them to explain why they recommend that product. They should be able to give you a clear answer with a scientific basis. For instance, does my hair need a protein conditioner or a moisturizing conditioner and why?

Good stylists should be able to give specific reasons to back up their suggestions.

In most salons, shampoos and conditioners are only the tip of the iceberg in the hair products department. The other items you may encounter are mousses, gels, waxes, pomades, spritzes, sprays, shiners, and so on. Whatever your stylist offers you as the greatest product on earth, make sure this person has shown you a real need for it. In other words, be crystal clear on why your hair needs to have that precious little bottle of goop. If it works well and is able to manipulate the hair to do exactly what you want it to do, then check the price and decide if it is worth it. In my hair-care line, I have a foaming pomade called Fommade. It sells for $15, which is certainly not cheap. The reason it's so expensive is because it's pressurized and contained in a rubber-coated glass bottle. It's costly to manufacture. When I demonstrate to a client what Fommade will do, however, the client usually agrees that it's worth it. Fommade is a magical styling tool that leaves the hair shiny and moldable. Clients love it, and it flies off the shelf. The price of a product is sometimes very much worth it, depending on the results. Make sure that you feel very good about your salon purchases by knowing specifically what the products will do.

With hair products, if you're on a budget, take baby steps. I would rather have a client buy just one good product, and really learn how to use it, than take home a whole bag of bottles and stick them on the shelf. Start with just one product designed to help you achieve your new style. On your next salon visit, you can add some other products that your stylist recommends. Take it slowly, and you'll learn more about how to manage your hair.

Skin Care

IN MY OPINION, here's where the real "Snake Oil" hides. The world of skin care is sometimes as mythical as the Fountain of Youth itself.

Wouldn't it be great to go to the salon for a facial and come home with a bag full of the latest miracle cures? Some salons jump on the dreamy bandwagon of promises to fight anti-aging and wrinkles. Here's where I get on my soapbox and start shouting. Listen carefully. *Many skin-care professionals spend more time attending product seminars than they have spent studying skin.* There is tremendous pressure in the salon industry to sell products. Many skin-care professionals get so wrapped up in selling you products that they actually begin to believe that what they're selling really works.

Now, let's be clear. A lot of products on the market do provide a real benefit when it comes to improving the appearance of the skin. I have my own skin-care line, and I'll be the first to tell you that these products are very effective. I get off the traditional skin-care boat, however, when the industry claims to provide unfounded and unrealistic solutions. Salon and skin-care professionals should be truthful about what a product will do. People seek out estheticians (those licensed in skin care) for answers about their skin. Estheticians are not trained in depth, as dermatologists are, but they can offer a lot more knowledge about skin than the salesperson at the cosmetics counter can. Estheticians have had a formal education focusing on skin. It is extremely important for the esthetician to adequately study and teach the basics about skin and how it functions. It is equally important not to recommend a product that defies the natural processes of skin. Be especially wary of any esthetician who claims to reverse and correct the aging process of the skin. To my knowledge, this cannot be done in a salon or by an esthetician. The only promises that should be made are to relieve the symptoms of aging skin or to make the skin look better. A medical doctor should perform medical procedures or invasive treatments for the aging process.

I'll address some treatments that estheticians perform later in this chapter, but first let's focus on products an esthetician may recommend. After seeing your skin up close and knowing a little about your history, an esthetician might suggest a skin-care routine. Some salons are big on the "skin-care ritual," whereby you must use several products daily to take care of your skin. Beware of their tendency to sell you a whole system. I am big on simplicity, especially if clients have never done anything to their skin except for using a bar of soap in the shower. The only real necessities, in my opinion, are a good cleanser for taking off your makeup, dirt, and perspiration; a good morning moisturizer with sun block or sunscreen; and an evening moisturizer with glycolic acid. Toners are effective in helping to give the skin an extra rinse after cleansing. Toners also help to tighten and close the pores, although they are not absolutely necessary to keep skin healthy. They contribute positively to the skin's appearance. I'll discuss skin care more in chapter 6, "Facials from Your Fridge."

If a client normally does a home facial, I may recommend a weekly scrub and/or a weekly mask. The extra time clients devote to themselves is always a good thing because it is gratifying psychologically, as well as beneficial for the skin. If a client seems unenthusiastic about going the extra mile for this home facial, then I just stick to the basics. I find that the realistic approach wins a lot of trust.

With skin-care products, it's very important to have the active ingredients explained, along with what benefits these will bring you. If the esthetician cannot successfully communicate what the product is designed to do, move on. Don't just buy it because it's on the counter. Second, listen carefully to the reasons for buying the product. It must deliver positive results, or you will probably be dissatisfied with it. Third, it must be reasonably priced. Skin-care products are nothing more than water, glycerin, emollients, and binders; very rarely, they're loaded with expensive miracle drugs. Products with alpha hydroxy acids will usually cost a little more. Products are worth more money if they contain no

SCENT-SITIVE

❖

Beware of skin-care products or makeup that is marketed as "Aromatherapy." Fragrances can be irritating, even if they are plant-derived. Skin-care products and makeup should not contain a lot of heavy scents. If you open a jar and the cream doesn't have a smell, it is usually more beneficial than a fragrant one for the skin.

artificial color or fragrance. Skin-care products should be relatively free of color and artificial fragrance anyway, because these can irritate certain types of skin.

Here are some warning signs to look out for when buying skin-care products:

1. Claims that are made about repairing or reversing the aging process. It can't be done in a salon.
2. The insistence that you buy the whole skin-care system, or it won't work.
3. Claims that a product will make your wrinkles disappear.
4. Claims that an esthetician knows as much about skin as a dermatologist or a plastic surgeon does. If estheticians did, they would probably be in these professions.
5. Claims that a product will cure chronic acne. I never waste a teenager's time while scars might be developing; I send the teen to a reputable dermatologist. (Light cases of acne are treatable with certain salon products.)
6. Claims that a product will make your skin firmer. There are some new products being developed that claim to restore skin's elasticity, but the jury is still out, along with FDA approval. At this time, the only aid in helping skin's firmness besides plastic surgery is facial exercises.
7. Estheticians trying to sell you a moisturizer because your skin is "dehydrated." Everyone's skin is dehydrated at the surface; that's the way skin works. As the dying skin cells travel up to the surface, they dry out and are sloughed off. Dehydration isn't an unusual or specialized problem that you may have. Decide whether you need a moisturizer by how your skin feels.
8. Cleansers that contain glycolic acid or alpha hydroxy acids. They are a waste of money because the acid ingredients are washed down the drain before they have a chance to work. Acid ingredients should remain on the skin to be effective and are only effective in moisturizers.

If you speak frankly to your esthetician about wanting to purchase products that really work, you may be surprised at the response. A good esthetician will be knowledgeable and will recommend only items that you need. Remember that skin care is usually overpriced. Don't get seduced into thinking that the higher the price, the better the product. I have seen ineffective junk put in a beautiful glass jar and packaged in an artistic box, then marked up to $85. I used to work at a salon in the most exclusive part of my hometown. I discovered that people would pay twice as much for products there, just because they were in the high-rent district. Good skin care is not necessarily expensive.

Be wary of skin-care lines that are too complicated. Many skin-care lines are multifaceted; their salesmen try to get you to believe that they can customize a system just for you. Skin isn't really that complicated, other than being normal, dry, or oily. In my opinion, the simpler a line is, the better.

Finally, I want to focus on the new "percentage game" that skin-care lines play with the consumer. Some skin-care lines charge more money for products that contain a higher percentage of an ingredient, particularly glycolic acid. For instance, a cream with 10 percent glycolic acid costs $30, but if you buy the jar with 20 percent glycolic acid, the price jumps to $40. In the first place, raising the percentage of glycolic acid from 10 to 20 percent would increase costs to the manufacturer by only pennies a jar. The increase to you is highway robbery—unthinkable, in my book. With any glycolic or alpha hydroxy acid cream, the percentage is unimportant compared to the pH level. Follow me on this; I'll tell you something that even most estheticians don't know. The amount of acid put in any cosmetic product can be diminished if it is added to an alkaline base cream. It's true that acid-based creams are effective in making skin look better because they chemically exfoliate the skin. This loosening of the surface cells will make the skin softer and appear younger. Just adding higher percentages of acids doesn't necessarily mean the cream is at an effective pH level to do a good job. That's why it is imperative to ask the pH level of any acid-based cream. Most estheticians will respond to this question with a blank stare because, usually, they don't know. For a glycolic acid cream to have a positive effect, it must be more acidic than the skin's natural state. Most skin has a pH range of 4.5 to 5.5. I recommend acid creams that are between 3.2 and 3.8, to be effective as a treatment. I'm not suggesting that you march around a salon with pH testing paper; I just want you to know a little about pH levels so that you don't waste your money. The next time an esthetician tries to entice you by boasting about the high percentage of acid in a cream, give her the "pH inquisition." You'll quickly discover what that person knows about how acid creams work.

Natural Alternatives

IF ALL THIS skin-care mumbo jumbo gives you a headache, you're not alone. One of the main reasons I developed my *Natural Beauty* TV show was to give people an alternative to the cosmetics skin-care hype. Just ahead are my natural skin-care recipes, in chapter 6, "Facials from Your Fridge." I hope you'll be enlightened by this more natural approach.

Body Care

MOST OF THE PRODUCTS in the massage and body-care department appeal to our emotions and noses. Aromatherapy is hugely popular in salons and day spas and for good reason. Aromatherapy offers a whole new dimension to self-therapy and relaxation. Most of the products are very straightforward and don't require a lot of discussion, such as candles, essential oils, and body oils. Be aware that massage oils are usually made from simple ingredients and should not cost much. You'll be amazed at how easily you can create your own spa line at home (see chapter 13, "Spa at Home").

Essential oils may be priced differently from salon to salon, so shop around and look for the best price. Pure essential oils are just that and should not vary from brand to brand. They should not be sold at inflated prices unless they are packaged in an unusual way.

Other items found in the body-care department are body scrubs, mitts, shower and bath washes, and soaps. I always like to educate people about using bar soap. I can't endorse soap bars, even for washing hands, for a few reasons. Soap bars are made of alkaline detergents, sometimes lye, and can be very harsh to the skin. The fats that are used to form soap bars leave a residue on the skin, much as they leave a residue on the sides of your bathtub, shower, or sink. I remember going on a camping trip when I was a teenager and forgetting to pack the shampoo. I used a bar of soap, as I'm sure many of you have in a pinch. Remember how your hair felt? The hair never felt clean because of the oils from the fats found in bar soap. Some bar soaps even have waxes in them. I know that many of you love soap, and there is a big market for soap lovers. Some people believe in vegetable and glycerin-based soaps. I have made my own soap and tested many bar soaps in search of a good one. Still, as a skin-care professional, I can't endorse bar soap because of the film it leaves. Sorry; I hope you will try body cleaners in a liquid form and see if you like the way your skin feels.

Body scrubs are abundant in most salons and day spas, and I love them. Make sure you like the feel of the scrub you purchase and that it isn't too soft or too gritty. A good body scrub should be affordable. If you are considering a fancy, expensive one, don't bother. I'll teach you how to make some great recipes in just a few chapters.

There is "Snake Oil" in the body-care department of many salons and day spas. Beware of any product that claims to repair or prevent stretch marks or cellulite. I get a little disgusted at products that make such claims. Stretch marks are like wrinkles. They form deep in the dermis and are permanent until treated by a doctor. If skin could repair itself where there is a stretch mark, then plastic surgeons would be

Do Play Dumb

When someone is "pitching" a product to you, pretend you are a four-year-old and ask "why?" repeatedly until you get a crystal-clear answer about the reason you need the product.

partially out of business. The interesting thing about stretch marks is that often they are not even formed specifically because of stretching, but because of hormone levels that are secreted in females at the time of pregnancy or puberty. Some women escape puberty and pregnancy without one single stretch mark. Others are not so lucky. Rubbing a miracle cream on the skin during pregnancy will not accomplish a thing except give you false hope. Once a stretch mark has formed, it will fade slightly over time, but a cream will not make it go away. Invest your money in a consultation with a plastic surgeon, instead of in a fancy jar.

Cellulite that forms in the fat tissue is simply a fancy name for fat. I have never found a cream or solution that you could rub on the skin that will go into the fat layer and break up cellulite. Many people will try to sell you on this idea. There would be a lot fewer lumpy legs walking around if that were true. Many creams and gels have an ingredient in them that manufacturers claim will transverse through the tissues and miraculously treat cellulite. Don't believe them. The way to solve this age-old problem is to eat properly and exercise. You probably knew that already, but wanted to cling to the hope of a cure in a jar.

Snake-Oil Salon Services

SOMETIMES I'M A LITTLE embarrassed to be in the salon industry when I hear about the crazy products and services that salons offer to consumers. I guess I just have to take things with a grain of salt and offer what I believe in. Here's a look at services that I feel you should be wary of.

TANNING BOOTHS

In the salon business we're supposed to promote looking good and practicing healthful skin care, yet a huge corner of the salon and day spa market still promotes and profits from tanning booths. To me, it's like having a cigarette machine in the lobby of a hospital. With all that we know about the ill effects of tanning, such as skin cancer and wrinkles, it boggles my mind that tanning booths are even around. I cannot in good conscience encourage tanning booths or even sunbathing. I've had girls younger than 20 in my facial chair, sporting the wrinkles of a 40-year-old, who ask me to recommend skin care. Please take a good look at any salon or spa that tries to sell you tanning services. There is nothing healthy or beautiful about what lies ahead for people who tan. You can never recover the damage that ultraviolet rays create in your skin. No amount of skin care can reverse the ill effects.

Alternatives to the tanning booth are available in many salons, in the form of a topical cream. I have used and promoted self-tanning creams for years. We offer a sunless tanning service in my day spa. The results look great and are very safe. The client can even use the product at home. I'll admit that having a richer color to the skin makes us feel healthier. We associate a tan with being healthy. Try and consider getting the bronze look in a healthful way with a self-tanning cream.

Body Wraps

Here's an interesting service offered in salons today. Some businesses solely offer body wraps, claiming that body wraps will get rid of body fat without exercise. Several different types of body wraps are commonly practiced. One type I approve of, but the other I don't. I'll address the negative one first.

Compression Wrapping

A compression body wrap will effectively cause your body to shrink. One hour after you enter a salon for a compression wrap, your clothes will definitely be baggy. Instant magic, but here's what happens in a compression wrap. The body is wrapped fairly tightly in ace bandages that have been steeped in a solution designed to extract the fat and toxins from the body. For the next half hour to an hour, you lie there and relax, to give the wrap a chance to work. Some wrap systems have clay infused into the solution the bandages are soaked in. As the clay dries, the bandages shrink, compressing the body fat. When the bandages are removed, Voila, you are thinner, tighter, smaller, and so forth. You get up and put on your clothes, smiling. It's a miracle, right? Wrong. The only thing that happened is that the adipose tissue was temporarily compressed. Your body will most likely return to its normal state a few hours later. You may have lost a little bit of bulk in the tissues by perspiring, but that could have been achieved by sitting around at home in sweats or exercising. The real danger in this kind of body wrap is not difficult to understand. Think about what happens if you wrap a rubber band tightly around your finger. The circulation is cut off. Now, admittedly, a body wrap doesn't cut off your circulation to that degree, but wrapping the whole body in tight bandages for an hour is a bit risky to the circulatory system. Since shedding unwanted pounds has everything to do with good circulation, the wrap is working in the wrong direction. Use your common sense when it comes to this type of wrap.

Loose Herbal or Seaweed Wrapping

Other body wraps that can be beneficial are loose herbal or seaweed wraps. I have had great results from a seaweed wrap, even after just one session. The body is loosely wrapped in herb-soaked sheets or plastic after a seaweed solution is applied. You usually lie still under a warm blanket for 30 minutes to an hour. It can be very relaxing and peaceful. The biggest effect from this type of wrap is water loss through perspiration. Some companies that sell wrap products boast that the seaweed and herbal solutions will promote extra perspiration and stimulate circulation. Try a wrap of this type for yourself to see whether it's worth it. A wrap should be done in tandem with diet and exercise. It should never be promoted as an alternative to diet and exercise. That is unrealistic.

PERMANENT MAKEUP

I'm one of the few salon professionals who believes that permanent makeup should be illegal unless performed by a physician. I strongly encourage you not to ever have it done. Permanent makeup is tattooing in the facial area to create a makeup look. Permanent makeup studios are cropping up all over the country. Consumers are trying the technique right and left. My fear is that most people don't know some of the hidden facts about permanent makeup and why they should avoid it.

First of all, it may shock you to learn that in many states, no certification is required to administer permanent makeup. In other words, anyone can pick up a tattoo gun and start performing the service. I think most people believe that permanent makeup artists have been licensed or at least tested by some government body. Surely, one can't just hang up a shingle and begin sticking dye around my eyeball or inject my lips with pink pigments. The answer is, yes, they can—and they do. In my early days as an esthetician, every week I received a pamphlet advertising a weekend seminar teaching how to apply permanent makeup. Later, I just received catalogs for supplies, such as the guns and inks. Anyone could pick up the supplies and just do it. If you walk into a permanent makeup studio, you may not know whether the person doing the service is a first-timer or very experienced. *There usually is no government certification or license for this service.*

In addition to that, you can probably raise some obvious cautionary flags on your own. The cleanliness of the needles, the skill of the artist, your sensitivity to the dyes being placed under your skin, and, of course, the permanence of the procedure.

My biggest reason for trying to talk you out of this service is because of the way it looks. As a makeup artist, I have done thousands of faces. I have detected permanent makeup on every woman who had it done. In my opinion, it doesn't look real. Because the dyes are placed under the skin, the makeup has a strange-looking quality. I realize that it sounds great to be able to wake up every day and not have to put on makeup, but the trade-off of looking unnatural is not worth it.

The name *permanent makeup* is a bit of false advertising. The dyes placed under the skin spread out and travel over time. Have you ever seen a tattoo on a serviceman over 60 years old? Tattoos get blurry and thicker over time. Can you imagine what will happen to your new charcoal eyebrows in about 30 years? A lady in her seventies came to me once to get advice about her eyebrows. She'd had them done in the early 1980s at one of the first permanent makeup studios in Las Vegas. Twenty years later, I sat there in shock over what to do for her. The brows had grown to twice their original size and were a light blue color. The charcoal ink had traveled and lightened to a paler color. The best I could do was try to conceal them with heavy foundation and show her how to recreate them with makeup. I encouraged her to see a plastic surgeon who specialized in tattoo removal.

When permanent makeup came out on the market, it was originally performed by doctors to line the eyes and replace eyeliner. The doctors generally stopped offering the service as salons took over. It was more trouble than it was worth for the docs. There are numerous cases of people with serious complications because of allergic reactions to the dyes. I witnessed a story on *60 Minutes* in which one woman had such a severe reaction that she had to have her permanent eyeliner removed with a laser. She lost all of her eyelashes in the process. If you had hoped to have this service done, I encourage you to reconsider.

Permanent tattooing for breast reconstruction is valuable to restore the appearance of nipples. I can also recommend permanent makeup to fill in small places in the hairline to conceal scars where hair will not grow. Other than that, I remain on my quest to discourage the practice. I know that many permanent makeup artists may be very experienced and skilled at their jobs, but I will withhold my endorsement until a regulatory board is established to ensure consumer safety.

MICRODERMABRASION

As the 1990s neared an end, companies rushed to manufacture machines to deliver the new Fountain of Youth in salons. Microdermabrasion was born. Microdermabrasion is a service that exfoliates the top layers of skin cells, using a machine that works like a sandblaster. Miniature crystals are blown onto the skin and vacuumed up quickly, taking surface cells along. I was intrigued at this new service and called a manufacturer for a demonstration. My findings were so negative I decided to forego the purchase of the machine.

The microdermabrasion treatment is sold as a package. Many salons promote it as a lunchtime peel. Clients can go to the salon on their lunch hour, receive the treatment, then go back to work with just a little redness. After five to 10 treatments, you're supposed to see a dramatic difference in the condition of your skin. Each treatment averages $150, so your total investment can end up costing over $1,000.

The results are supposed to include a finer skin texture; softer, less noticeable wrinkles; and a lightening of age spots.

Since I don't offer this treatment in my salon, I can't give you real examples of success stories. I can only give you my impression of the treatment. When I tested it, I had a representative come to my salon with the $15,000 machine to give me a treatment. My first red flag was when the rep put on a surgical mask. She explained that it was advisable for the operator to wear it so that the crystals would not get into her lungs. *What about the client's lungs?* I thought. The machine spits out a constant stream of fine crystals all over the client's skin. That did not sit well with me because, unless the client holds his or her breath, the crystals will probably drift into the client's lungs.

I found the treatment to be far from painless; it was very uncomfortable. As the wand grazes over the skin, it smarts. The shock was after the treatment. I had a very uneven pattern of red scratches all over my face where the head of the wand had passed. A few days later, the scratches had faded, but there was absolutely no change in my skin. The procedure was hardly worth the $150 charge.

What you should know about microdermabrasion is that you could perform the equivalent yourself by simply rubbing a gritty substance on your skin long enough to achieve a stinging sensation. The high-tech machine leads people to believe that something magical is taking place. You get nothing more from microdermabrasion than you would from standing in a sandstorm. It is simply a deeper method of skin exfoliation. Don't be fooled by the machine or the high price of the treatments. Don't rush out to get this service just because a friend of yours did, and you feel like you're missing out on a new skin miracle.

By the way, there are many used microdermabrasion machines listed in the "for sale" sections of the salon trade magazines I receive weekly. This tells me that some salons may be dropping this service, which may be due to the lack of clients who want it.

If you're still enthusiastic about trying this procedure, ask a lot of questions. It might be a good idea to get a list of clients who have had it done and ask them about the results. You may save yourself hundreds of dollars.

ELECTRICAL FACIAL TONING

This service is offered to tighten and tone facial muscles. The procedure is relatively simple. Electrodes are placed on the face, and an electrical current is used to stimulate muscle contractions. This method is effective; it's used in physical therapy all the time to help stimulate muscles to prevent atrophy. The effect is temporary, however. To perpetuate the improved tone in the facial muscles, you must continue to get treatments. The service is a little addictive. For the price of one or two of these treatments, you could purchase your own machine for home use. A few facial toning machines are out on the market, none that I have tried or would endorse. I have seen a few infomercials that sell facial toning masks. Try these products at your own risk. I just want you to be aware that there are machines made for home use.

In the state of California, where I live, licensed salons are forbidden to use electric currents to stimulate muscle activity. I agree with this law, because at this time, training isn't provided in local schools. You may receive a treatment by someone with inexperienced hands. Be careful if you choose to have this service.

CELLULITE MASSAGERS

There are now machines on the market designed to treat cellulite, the lumpy fat that gathers on some people's thighs and buttocks. Basically, the machine utilizes a suction technique to massage the skin. Proponents of this treatment swear by the results. My instincts tell me to be a little skeptical. Massage does help to stimulate circulation, and that may be a small part of anyone's weight-loss program. I feel that a good body massage would probably deliver as much benefit as this type of machine. Use your common sense, or ask for a free demonstration of the treatment.

OXYGEN FACIAL TREATMENTS

Did you know that many salons give facials by employing an oxygen tank? The treatment room looks like an intensive care unit. Oxygen facials use pure oxygen, straight out of a pressurized tank, delivered directly to the face during the service. The theory is that pure oxygen will improve the condition of the skin, and many estheticians believe this to be true. This idea may have come from the practice that developed in the last decade for burn patients. Doctors discovered that the skin healed more quickly for burn patients when pure oxygen was administered topically.

The administration of pure oxygen during a facial is speculative. I believe that it gives little or no benefit. Your skin is nourished from the bloodstream. The skin's main function is to offer protection from the elements. It is an effective barrier unless the skin is broken. My best recommendation is to forego the oxygen and save yourself some money.

My Message

MY WARNINGS ABOUT "Snake Oil" are intended to save you money and give you insight into treatments and products that warrant a second look. Listen to your own intuition when pulling out your wallet to chase the dream of beauty, whether it be in a bottle or a treatment room. Everyone has a limit when spending money to look good. Use the money in your budget wisely so that you receive the optimum results. Remember, above all, that the price of a product or treatment doesn't necessarily correlate with the results. You'll save yourself a lot of disappointment if you spend your dollars on products and services that bring visible changes. The benefits should be clear and favorable. Don't buy "Snake Oil" for the sake of spending and don't help promote "Snake Oil" to others to help justify your purchase. Be an ambassador of common sense. You'll feel better from the inside out and ultimately look better, too!

· 5 ·
Inner Beauty

"Taking joy in life is a woman's best cosmetic." ROSALIND RUSSELL

A FRIEND TOLD me that his father once advised him, "If you can accept criticism the same way you accept compliments, you will develop a thankful spirit." Inner strength comes from inner peace; therefore, when you display an inner beauty, your soul will look fabulous. Though you may not look gorgeous all the time, it doesn't mean you can't feel good about yourself by focusing on your inner beauty. Cosmetics, clothes, diet, and exercise can help you look good, but self-esteem and peace will help you put inner beauty as a daily priority in life. Once you're in touch with your own inner beauty, you'll realize an improvement in how you look and feel.

Inner beauty transcends physical appearance. A certain countenance will be revealed through sparkling eyes, a winning smile, and a joyous spirit. Renowned psychologist Dr. Joyce Brothers says, "A strong positive self-image is the best possible preparation for success. A woman's warmth, righteousness, and virtue make her beautiful. Inner and outer beauty is influenced by happiness or lack of it. Unhappiness will be read on her face, no matter how much makeup she is wearing."

Let go of negative feelings and self-doubt and concentrate on seeking happiness. Happiness doesn't happen to us as a result of someone or something. Happiness is a choice.

Happy thoughts are more effective than expensive salon treatments. Once you've discovered your inner beauty, it will appear on your face and you will take on a softer impression. How pretty you are perceived by others may be determined by your attitude.

Attitude

HAVE YOU EVER NOTICED that some people are happy no matter what? Over the years I have met individuals who have a positive attitude 24 hours a day, seven days a week. The happiness that radiates from these people rarely happens because of external influences like money, social status, or material possessions. A happy spirit comes from an internal drive, a drive to be happy. The real beauty is that this drive becomes contagious. When we are in the presence of a happy person, it is uplifting. I refer to this type of happy person as a "spark plug."

When a "spark plug" walks into my salon and sits in my styling chair before the mirror, it's sometimes difficult to find what needs improving. That person simply looks great. Conversely, when an unhappy or negative person sits in front of the mirror, all the talent I can muster seldom brings beautiful results. No amount of hairspray can perk up a grumpy disposition. No magical makeup palette can beautify a frown.

Unfortunately, you can't hide the outer effects of your attitude. It shows on your face. It can be seen in your eyes. It can be telegraphed by your facial expressions.

Improving your attitude should be a constant, daily part of your beauty regime. Once you are convinced of how important attitude is, the pathway to a better attitude is easier to follow.

ATTITUDE ADJUSTMENT

The word *attitude* is described as a way of thinking. Our way of thinking can be positive or negative and can jump back and forth rather quickly. Keeping their attitude on an even keel and in the positive mode comes naturally for some, but is difficult for others. To strive for consistency in your positive attitude, it may be helpful to analyze which forces can inhibit a cheerful attitude.

AN INNER MAKEOVER

When a negative thought creeps into your brain, replace it with a positive one. That's the beauty of the mind, we can change it at any time.

Black Clouds

AFTER 20 YEARS OF working closely with thousands of people, I have heard everyone's problems in the salon. People tend to unload on their hairstylists. I didn't sign up to be a pseudopsychologist, but ended up listening to the problems of others. I have identified what I call the "Five Enemies" of a great attitude. I'm sure there are others, but these seem to be the most common:

1. Stress
2. Worry
3. Jealousy
4. Self-Doubt
5. Self-Pity

STRESS

When I ask a frowning person, "What's wrong?" the number one answer I get is, "I'm so stressed!" or "I'm handling a lot of stress!" When I dig a little deeper to be polite, I discover that the stress in many people's lives is totally controllable or avoidable altogether. Here are some typical scenarios and possible solutions:

*P*ROBLEM: Time stress—I'm always late for work or school!

*S*OLUTION: Get up 15 minutes earlier. Convince yourself that you need more time to get there and make it a habit.

*P*ROBLEM: The boss is always on my back!

*S*OLUTION: Have a heart-to-heart with your supervisor or boss to better define this person's expectations. Make a plan to work toward meeting your boss's expectations. Follow up with more meetings to improve communications. Most job stress is due to misunderstandings.

*P*ROBLEM: The household is chaotic because of children, chores, pets, and schedules.

*S*OLUTION: Have a family meeting to get better organized. Make it a goal for everyone to simplify and slow down.

*P*ROBLEM: Money issues are stressful.

*S*OLUTION: Money or the lack of it seems to control people's lives. Don't let it! Consider living with less money. Adopt a simpler way of life. Live in a more modest home. Drive a less expensive car. Acquire less "stuff." Plan activities that don't cost a lot of money. Instead of going to the movies, go to a free museum. Go to the park for a picnic instead of to a restaurant. Play a game of ball with your child instead of buying that new video game cartridge. You get the picture. All the things that we think we need in order to be happy are being funded by more stress, eroding our happiness.

*P*ROBLEM: Commuting in traffic is making me crazy!

*S*OLUTION: Live near work or work near where you live. This is such a simple concept that Europeans have practiced it for years. It's one reason Europeans have more leisure time to enjoy themselves.

They also use public transportation, giving them more time to relax or read during a commute. Take a deep breath and get to work more efficiently. Spending hours on the freeway could be better spent with your family and friends. Time to yourself or with loved ones is valuable. You may consider reevaluating your job's rate of pay to include the time it takes you to commute. When figuring in the commute time, you may find that the money you earn at work is less per hour. Taking a closer look at the rate of pay may encourage you to consider a change.

You may relate to these problems and solutions, or they may simply inspire you to address your own stressful situations. In my own life, alleviating stress is my priority, above making money to support a family. A peaceful, harmonious lifestyle is more important to me than anything else. Setting a goal to remove the source of stress is an important step. Next, write down what situations create stress in your life. Try to think of one or two possible solutions, even if they seem impossible to implement. Just by declaring on paper what causes your stress, you'll become more acutely aware of stress as it's brewing. As you begin to actively go through steps to eliminate the sources of stress, you'll feel more in control.

In the meantime, while you put your plan into action, consider some ways to impede or diminish stress.

For example, in a chaotic household, play classical music to soothe yourself and your children. Turn off the television more often. Open the curtains to let in light. Light candles to create a peaceful mood. Use relaxing aromatherapy oils on cotton balls scattered around the house. When the household activity level escalates, escape for a bath and a break.

In review, the three steps I recommend to alleviate stress are:

1. Identify the source of stress and write it down
2. Make a plan to remove the source of stress
3. Be creative with soothing yourself until you've eliminated the source

These three steps may seem elementary, but it really can be that easy. Suffering from continual stress is a changeable situation. You can choose to change.

WORRY

I recognize that most folks worry from time to time. I personally have never been a "worrier." It's an emotion I don't understand because I figured out long ago that worrying doesn't solve anything. I can't say any magic words to solve your tendency to worry, but I can tell you how I've learned to fend off worry.

Worry is a waste of time. Worry robs you of experiencing joy. Excessive worrying can paralyze you, preventing action. I see so many talented people with great ideas never progress because they talk themselves out of trying something, due to worry. I have a saying: "Never say, 'I think I can.' Say, 'I know I can,' then get to doing it."

There are two kinds of worry:

1. Worrying about things you can control
2. Worrying about things you can't control

If you find yourself worrying over something you have no control over, put the situation in a mental box, an imaginary crate or container; seal it; and place it somewhere on an imaginary shelf. If the situation you're worried about begins to affect your life, take it out of the box and deal with it. Until then, the box is sealed. You have too many other joyous things in your life to experience.

If you're worrying about something that you can control, transfer the "worry" to action. Write down the situation and what control you have over it. Make a step-by-step plan to reassure yourself what you will do to deal with the situation effectively. After writing out the plan, put the plan away in a desk drawer or file. Refer to it when the worry overtakes your mind. It will give you confidence to cope with it. Then you can free your mind up to enjoy other thoughts.

JEALOUSY

Jealousy is a strange emotion that is a real killer of inner beauty. When we become jealous of another human being, our entire attitude suffers and withers. Women can be very jealous creatures by nature, more so than men. Men are competitive, but don't react negatively when meeting up with a greater talent or another who is more handsome. When a woman views another woman as more stunning or beautiful than herself, she can experience admiration or jealousy. If the latter emotion takes over, the results are negativity, self-doubt, fear, and sometimes anger. All of these emotions will register outwardly. A jealous female will seldom radiate outer beauty.

Most of us have experienced jealousy at one time or another. Some women are literally crippled by it. It controls everything they think about and stems from low self-esteem. The good news about jealousy, which I learned from my days as a model, is that it's very easy to turn the negative feelings of jealousy into admiration. Admiration registers a positive quality with most people. It is almost synonymous with awe and wonder. When we admire someone, it usually means that we like them and want to be like them or possess the qualities that they possess. Jealousy, on the other hand, is a negative emotion that conveys dislike of another person.

When I auditioned for a modeling job and walked into a room of 40 gorgeous models, I initially surveyed the room and became overwhelmed with jealous feelings. I wanted to hate the other girls who were prettier than me and might rob me of the job. As time went on, I realized that they were humans just like me. Along with their attributes, they probably had their own jealousies and

PAY IT FORWARD

For an attitude boost, pass out at least three compliments to others every day. Be sincere in your comments and reap the benefits of the smiles you receive.

fears. As I felt the negative feelings creep in, I played a game. I looked at each girl and acted as if I was conducting the audition. I selected two or three things about each model that were great qualities of beauty. I viewed everyone in the room as teaching me a lesson about looking beautiful. I searched for a smile so that I could smile back. I tried to select the most appealing, the healthiest looking, or the sexiest in the group. In doing the talent search, I took myself out of the circle of comparison and I could soften my jealousy. I transformed jealousy to admiration and no longer killed my inner beauty with negativity. Here are some other effective ways to change a jealous nature to a positive attitude:

1. Try to admire the person that stirs up your jealous feelings.
2. If you find yourself jealous of the way somebody looks, study the things you feel jealous of and what that person presents that you can learn from—for example, makeup, hairstyle, and clothing.
3. When you find yourself jealous of someone, pretend that the person is your sister, brother, or best friend. Sometimes when you feel more connected to someone, your feelings of jealousy will soften.
4. Put yourself in the shoes of the person you're jealous of. Once you are in those shoes, realize that this person may be admiring you. Feel the admiration. By transferring the admiration to yourself, you might be better able to chase away your jealous feelings.

SELF-DOUBT

Self-doubt is an emotion we all battle many times every day. It is usually a fleeting emotion. Everyone needs motivation from time to time. That's why cheerleaders were created. You can be your own cheerleader. I often recall a saying that helps me combat self-doubt. "Who better than me to accomplish anything?" I also motivate myself by saying, "There are people less capable than me accomplishing that task!"

In other words, a lot of folks out there are setting out to accomplish many things, like owning a business, raising kids, teaching, athletics. If not you . . . then who? *The point is, you as much as anyone else can accomplish anything, you just have to decide that you can.* Self-doubt is self-defeating. It is the same as worrying; it robs you of the joy of trying. Face your fears, face your self-doubt, and *try.* If you don't try, you'll never know what you can accomplish. If you try and fail, at least you'll have a starting point to try and improve the next time around. Encourage yourself to ignore your self-doubt. Take a deep breath and move forward, even if it is with baby steps. You'll take bigger steps as time goes on.

Self-Pity

Self-pity takes a little more energy to overcome. Self-pity can result from a real trauma or circumstance that causes us to feel pain. The only problem with self-pity is that it occupies the brain and deprives you of the ability to move forward, beyond the events that caused you pain. For whatever reason that you pity yourself, try to concentrate on the *now.* Only by living with your current circumstances can you move on to enjoy life. Every day that you wake up, you have the ability to improve your life and grow beyond hurtful circumstances. Try playing a little game with yourself—I call it "The Middle Man." Know that in every aspect of your life you are always in the middle of a situation. In other words, there is always someone who has an easier life than you, but there is also someone who has a more difficult life than you. There is always someone richer than you and always someone poorer. Undoubtedly, someone out there is more gorgeous than you and someone is less attractive than you. Knowing that you are always in the middle may give you some relief when you judge yourself harshly.

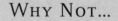

Why Not...

Buy yourself a small bouquet of flowers every once in a while, just because.

Inner Beauty Boosters

BESIDES ADJUSTING YOUR ATTITUDE, here are some other factors to boost your inner beauty:

1. Enthusiasm
2. Energy
3. Confidence
4. Healthful Living

ENTHUSIASM

Wake up every day committed to being enthusiastic. Your enthusiasm for life will boost that beauty within. Career. Parenting. Housework. How you take on tasks will reveal your interest in living life to the fullest. When you are enthusiastic, it will show in your smile. A winning smile can take years off your face. Let your eyes be expressive. They can reveal what you're thinking and feeling. Inner beauty can bring radiance to your eyes that no eyeliner, eye shadow, or mascara can match.

ENERGY

Most people believe that energy is a physical manifestation. I don't. I feel that it can be created with a positive will to be more energetic. It must come from within, just like enthusiasm. Creating your own energy can be an enjoyable endeavor. It's not about pumping yourself up with caffeine; just pump yourself up with an energetic spirit. Attack daily chores and tasks with a vengeance. See life as something worth seizing. Get small jobs done faster. Walk with a lighter gait. Stand up straight. Take the stairs. Pretend you are an Olympic athlete. Dream that you are an astronaut. Create your own Force and let the Force be with you.

CONFIDENCE

Confidence is a funny thing. It is a strong and powerful force that gives us the ability to conquer huge obstacles. Yet without it, we are sometimes crippled to accomplish even the smallest of tasks. Confidence is power, that's for sure. The power, however, comes from an internal power plant. My secret to confidence is pretending that I am a gifted actor. Whatever situation I am faced with, I play-act the part. I imagine what an actor would do to play the part. Then I become the actor and I act. The phrase "Fake it till you make it" has inspired me to tackle many things I've felt unsure about. Once I've set my mind, I follow through with a straight posture, an uplifted chin, and an award-winning smile. This is a case where the mind and body should work together to strengthen your confidence.

HEALTHFUL LIVING

Nothing can boost your inner beauty more than living healthfully. Eat right. Exercise. Love. Worship. Serve. Remind yourself daily that you must be in service to yourself. Give and receive massages. Play music. Laugh. Take naps. In a world

STOP!

Take a minute to look at the sunrise in the morning and the stars at night. During these two brief moments, recall a memorable occasion that made you happy.

that makes demands and issues deadlines daily, it is necessary for your physical and mental well-being to take time to do whatever makes you happy. Tell yourself you deserve it and you are worth it. Trade your evenings out for time at home to rest and relax. Get up earlier to start an exercise regime. Get your blood circulating. The amazing thing about increasing your physical activity is that you'll be less inclined to indulge in coffee, alcohol, cigarettes, and junk food. Your body will steer you into a better diet. Not only will you start to look more fit, your self-esteem will soar. The increase in your energy level will propel you into other positive daily habits. The greatest results will be a new vitality for life and a new appreciation of yourself.

These priorities are essential ingredients for inner beauty. How wonderful it is to *look* beautiful, but how life-changing it is to *feel* beautiful.

· 6 ·

Facials from Your Fridge

"Nature gives to every time and season some beauties of its own." CHARLES DICKENS

I WAS ABOUT 14 years old when I first read about mixing up egg whites and smearing them on your skin. I believe it was in an article in my older sister's *Seventeen* magazine. The egg whites were supposed to do something for your face, but at the time I didn't really know what. A few years later, my mom hosted a home demonstration for Mary Kay, and I gave myself my first facial, assisted by a nice lady in a pink suit. I knew that very day that I wanted a career in the skin-care business.

I managed to escape my teen years with clear skin, but hit acne problems in my twenties. Off to the cosmetics counter I went in search of the perfect remedy. I tried many over-the-counter products, but discovered no cure. Back to the kitchen I went, armed with knowledge from my college chemistry class. I revived the old egg whites recipe and started dabbling in others. I knew that my skin wasn't oily, but rather dry, so why was I breaking out? I soon discovered many natural and easy home-style skin-care secrets that actually worked to improve the quality of one's skin. (The recipes were also fun to make.)

Now you can discover what other women all around you have known for years—facials do make skin look and feel better and, maybe more important, they make us feel good about ourselves. There's something magical about taking an extra 10 or 20 minutes to practice a ritual for ourselves. It's relaxing and nurturing, inside and out.

The ritual is not limited to the face, by the way. You may start with the face, but I predict that you'll soon graduate to "body facials," which take care of the skin on your torso, arms, and legs. Most of us suffer from dry skin all over our bodies. This booklet will teach you how to make a simple body scrub to ease dry, dead skin.

Facial History

PEOPLE HAVE PAMPERED THEIR skin since the Egyptian days, rubbing everything from oils, crushed flower petals, ashes, honey, and mud all over the face and body. The modern-day facial has its roots in the European spa and is based on lubrication of the skin. Europeans believe that skin matures and dries out, creating wrinkles. Lubricating the skin with heavy oils and creams will soften or mask the aging process. In the 1980s a new age in skin care was born: the belief that the ill effects of photo-aging (sun damage) could be lessened by exfoliation, or rapid removal of the dead surface layer of skin cells. If the dead, dry layer of cells were swept away more frequently, new skin cells would be manufactured at a more rapid rate. This theory was the birth of renewed thinking in skin-care technology. *Exfoliation became the new key to fighting the effects of aging.*

My Personal Beliefs

I RECEIVED MY ESTHETICIAN license in 1986 during the advent of this new technology. I remember reading an article about fruit acids when I studied skin care. Scientists had discovered some amazing benefits for skin when applying alpha hydroxy acids, or AHAs. AHAs are a group of naturally occurring substances found in common foods. For instance, citric acid is from citrus fruits, tartaric acid is from grapes, lactic acid is from milk, and malic acid is from apples. The most revolutionary acid discovered for its ideal skin-care properties is glycolic acid, derived from sugar cane. Of all the AHAs, glycolic acid is the most effective, due to its small molecular size. Glycolic acid loosens the cement that holds the dry dead cells together in the stratum corneum, the top layer of skin. It speeds up surface cell exfoliation. The benefits include minimizing of fine lines, a smoother texture, and an increase in the hydration of the surface cells. Other fruits contain similar acids.

I soon began experimenting at home, as a class project. We were assigned to create a facial mask recipe and to justify the benefits in front of the class. Needless to say, I didn't stop at that one assignment. I have been working up recipes for the face and body for the last 15 years.

The following recipes will be fun and invigorating for you. At times, they may be a little messy. I hope you enjoy taking time for yourself and learning how to better take care of your skin.

How Skin Works

LET'S KEEP IT BASIC. Your skin covers the body mainly for protection. Because of its waterproof barrier, you can shower, swim, and walk in the rain without injuring the inside of your body. Your skin stays pliable because of its natural lubrication system. Oil is continually secreted by oil glands. Sweat glands produce perspiration to regulate your body temperature.

What Skin Benefits From
1. Daily cleansing
2. Daily toning
3. Daily moisturizing
4. Weekly exfoliation
5. Weekly acid treatment or specialty mask

I find that most people, especially women, tend to overdo it when it comes to skin care. First of all, I'll be the first to tell you that skin, for the most part, cleans itself. If it wasn't for makeup, pollution, and perspiration, you could keep your skin fairly clean and healthy with a washcloth and warm water.

Know Your Skin Type

IT'S IMPORTANT TO KNOW what kind of skin you have because many of the recipes in this booklet are designed to tackle certain types of skin issues. Many recipes will be marked with symbols to help you determine what type of skin they are designed for:

$\mathcal{N}$ = Normal

$\mathcal{D}$ = Dry

$\mathcal{O}$ = Oily

$\mathcal{S}$ = Sensitive

NORMAL SKIN ($\mathcal{N}$)

Most people have normal skin, but I spend a lot of time convincing women and men of that. Normal skin will usually seem shiny by noon each day. Some people think this shininess means that their skin is actually oily, but try to think of these criteria in determining whether you have oily or normal skin: Oily skin is usually shiny an hour after cleansing and may be accompanied by blackheads, acne, or both. Normal skin will have the presence of a shine, but the condition of the skin is clear, without the presence of blackheads or acne.

Dry Skin (𝒟)

There is usually no mistaking dry skin. The skin feels tight almost all the time, it is never shiny, and it may sometimes even have a flaky look. Dry skin will usually age more quickly, so those with dry skin should be especially aware of sun exposure.

Oily Skin (𝒪)

Oily skin gets shiny almost immediately after midmorning and may be accompanied by acne or blackheads. Some people with oily skin don't suffer from any problems that are associated with oily skin; they just have to tolerate the shine. The good news about oily skin is that it tends to age more gracefully.

Sensitive Skin (𝒮)

Sensitive skin is usually identified as fair- to medium-toned skin that gets red or irritated due to stimulation associated with sunlight, exfoliation, or cosmetic preparations. Most people with oily skin do not have sensitive skin. Oily skin tends to be fairly sturdy and does not react in a sensitive nature. Normal and dry skin can sometimes be delicate and fall under the sub-classification of *sensitive.* People with sensitive skin usually can identify the problem easily. They tend to get sunburned easily and will react adversely to harsh soaps and cosmetics. If you have sensitive skin, avoid the use of extra gritty exfoliators and strong acid treatments.

Your Skin-Care Routine

THE BEST COMPLEXIONS I'VE seen belonged to people with two things in common:

1. Good genetics
2. Consistent skin-care habits

Getting into the swing of a regular skin-care routine will serve you well; you'll see and feel a difference. I'll give you some ideas about home "potions" that are easy to put together with the most basic of kitchen staples. Some of you will be very faithful about sticking to your routine. You may be so enthused about these recipes that you use them exclusively. Some of you will mix them in with commercial products you already buy. Whatever the case, remember that consistency is the best strategy when it comes to results. Even on my lazy nights, I always remove my makeup with a basic cleanser.

NIGHT ROUTINE

At the end of the day, I recommend a gentle cleansing with a mild cleanser and warm water and washcloth for exfoliation. Apply a toner next, especially if you have oily skin. It will give the skin an extra rinse and help to tighten the pores. Following the toner, apply a lightweight moisturizer. I prefer commercially prepared moisturizers to the homemade ones because they generally contain special ingredients that have optimum benefits for your skin. Your evening moisturizer should contain glycolic acid. (Your morning moisturizer should contain a sun block.)

MORNING ROUTINE

In the morning, if you've cleansed your face properly the night before, you'll simply need to rinse your face in the shower or sink with good old H_2O. Follow with a toner for a fresh feeling and to tighten up pores. Finish with your morning moisturizer with sun block.

WEEKLY ROUTINE

Once a week, your skin will benefit from an exfoliating scrub or mask. This process will help clear the surface of the skin of dry cells and give your skin a softer, less-wrinkled appearance.

After your weekly exfoliation, your skin and your mental health will further benefit from a treatment mask, designed to target any special problem you may have with your skin. In this chapter, you'll learn how to make some terrific, beneficial masks, scrubs, cleansers, and toners.

Basic Ingredients for the Whole Family

WHEN I GO TO the grocery store, I always stock up on the following items for a full array of skin-care potions. Some of them are perishable and need to be purchased often. Many of them have a longer shelf life.

Pantry Items	Refrigerator Items	Drugstore Items
Baking Soda	Avocado	Beeswax Pellets
Canola Oil	Eggs	Epsom Salts
Chamomile Tea	Lemons	Isopropyl Alcohol
Cornmeal	Margarine	Milk of Magnesia
Cornstarch	Mayonnaise	(unflavored)
Cream of Wheat	Milk	Witch Hazel
Gelatin (unflavored)	Oranges	
Green Tea	Papaya	
Honey	Sour Cream	
Iodized Salt	Strawberries	
Oat Bran	Tomatoes	
Oatmeal	Yogurt (plain)	
Pectin		
Powdered Milk		
Tomato Paste		
Tomato Sauce		
Sugar		

From these simple ingredients, you will be able to concoct many recipes for your skin-care routine, including cleansers, scrubs, masks, and acid treatments. Ready? Here we go!

Cleansers

REMEMBER, WE ARE PREPARING a cleanser to clean the skin nightly of makeup, dirt, and perspiration. You can prepare this cleanser nightly or you can mix up a larger batch and store in the refrigerator.

There will be times when you'll want a smooth, gentle cleanser and other times when you'll want a deep cleanser. We will classify the "heavy" cleansers that deep clean and exfoliate as "scrubs."

BASIC CLEANSER FOR ALL SKIN TYPES *NDOS*

1 TEASPOON YOGURT

½ TEASPOON HONEY

*M*ix together in a small cup and massage all over the face. Rinse and remove with warm water and a washcloth.

The lactic acid in yogurt is ideal for skin. Honey is the only food found in nature that bacteria doesn't grow in. That's why a jar of honey can be left out without refrigeration. Honey is beneficial for antibacterial cleansing.

BASIC CLEANSER FOR DRY SKIN *D*

1 TEASPOON YOGURT

½ TEASPOON MAYONNAISE

½ TEASPOON FINELY GROUND OATMEAL

SEASONAL FACE FOOD

Store your yogurt and honey cleanser in a squeeze bottle in the refrigerator (a restaurant-style, plastic ketchup bottle is perfect for storing). It will be a refreshing treatment at the end of a warm day to remove makeup and perspiration. In the wintertime, squeeze the cleanser into a small paper cup and microwave for 10 to 20 seconds for a warm relaxing treatment.

*G*rind the oatmeal in a food processor. It's convenient to grind up a large batch and store it for future use. Mix all ingredients together and massage all over the face. Remove with warm water and a washcloth. The oatmeal acts as a skin softener, while the oils in the mayonnaise moisturize the skin.

Basic Cleanser for Oily Skin *O*

1 TEASPOON YOGURT

1 EGG WHITE

1 TEASPOON MILK OF MAGNESIA (UNFLAVORED)

*M*ix together and massage all over the face. Remove with warm water and a washcloth. If skin is very oily and acne is present, allow the cleanser to dry for five minutes before removing. This recipe makes enough cleanser to last three or four days. Simply store in a small plastic container and keep refrigerated.

Deep Cleanser *NDOS*

Use this after heavy sports when you've perspired a lot or for nights when you've worn a lot of makeup. The oatmeal helps to soften skin and the oils will act as a solvent for heavy makeup and clogged pores.

½ CUP OATMEAL

3 TO 4 DROPS SWEET ALMOND OIL OR CANOLA OIL

1 TABLESPOON MILK

1 EGG WHITE

*G*rind up oatmeal in a food processor. Add remaining ingredients and blend and massage all over the face and neck for two to three minutes. It's a little messy, so bend over the sink while you massage it in. Rinse with a washcloth and warm water. This cleanser will leave the skin very clean and soft.

Toners

TONERS SHOULD BE APPLIED immediately after the cleansing step. Toners are made of liquid ingredients designed to rinse the skin, remove oils, and tighten up pores. They are an important second step to the cleansing process. Never rinse off a toner; just let the liquid evaporate on your skin. The evaporation of the toner is what helps contract the pores. Here are my favorite toner recipes:

Witch Hazel $\mathcal{N}$ $\mathcal{D}$ $\mathcal{O}$: Apply plain old witch hazel straight from the bottle to the face with a cotton ball. Let it evaporate. You may pour the witch hazel into a bottle with a spray so it can be sprayed directly on the skin after cleansing. Avoid the eye area.

Lemon Juice Toner $\mathcal{O}$: Squeeze half a lemon and add it to one cup of water. Strain off pulp and seeds and pour into a small plastic bottle, shake well, and apply to the face with a cotton ball. Use a spray top on your bottle to spray the toner on the skin. Let evaporate. An added benefit to the lemon juice toner is that the citric acid helps to fade age and brown spots over time. Store in the refrigerator between uses.

Chamomile Tea $\mathcal{N}$ $\mathcal{D}$ $\mathcal{S}$: Steep a chamomile tea bag in hot water. After the tea has cooled, add an equal part of fresh water. Pour into a plastic bottle and apply to the skin with a cotton ball. You may choose a spray top for dispensing directly on the skin.

Green Tea $\mathcal{N}$ $\mathcal{D}$ $\mathcal{O}$ $\mathcal{S}$: This is my new favorite for all skin types. Steep a green tea bag in 1 cup of hot water, then let it cool. Add 1 cup of fresh water and pour into a small plastic bottle. Apply to the face with a cotton ball or spray it on.

> ### SIMPLE CLEANING
>
> ❦
>
> *Remember that water is the best natural cleanser of all. Dampen a washcloth and microwave for 30 seconds to 1 minute. After applying your natural cleanser, rinse off with your warm washcloth. The cloth will aid in exfoliation.*

Facial Exfoliation

EXFOLIATION IS THE SECRET to beautiful smooth skin. When you go to a salon for a professional facial, the most noticeable treatment that is performed is a scrub or peel treatment. These very expensive treatments can be duplicated by my blends made right in your kitchen. Try to do an exfoliating treatment at least twice a week. Don't overdo them, or you'll irritate your skin!

Gentle Scrub 𝒩 𝒟 𝒪 𝒮: Mix 1 egg yolk with 1 tablespoon of oat bran or oatmeal (the instant kind is better). You may add a teaspoon of warm water for a smoother consistency. Scoop up the preparation with your fingers and massage all over the face and neck. Massage in small circular motions for two to three minutes. Rinse with warm water. Follow with a toner and moisturizer of your choice. This scrub is very mild, not gritty.

Sugar Scrub for Aging Skin 𝒩 𝒟: Blend 1 tablespoon sugar with 1 tablespoon vegetable oil. Massage all over the face and neck for two to three minutes. Rinse with warm water and a washcloth to eliminate the oil residue. Follow with a toner of your choice and moisturize.

This scrub will impress you with how well it works. There is a commercial product just out on the market that has sugar and olive oil as the only ingredients. The cosmetics company that manufactures this is one of the giants. It is charging $32 for a 10-ounce jar. The previous recipe costs pennies to make!

Cornmeal Scrub for Acne 𝒪: Mix 1 tablespoon of cornmeal with 1 egg white; add a little bit of warm water, if necessary,

---

❀❀❀❀❀❀❀❀❀❀❀❀❀

NATURAL TONER PADS

Purchase gauze squares from the first aid section of your grocery store and place them in a plastic container with a lid. Pour your favorite natural toner over the pads to soak them. The pads are ready to use at any time for facial toning after cleansing.

❀❀❀❀❀❀❀❀❀❀❀❀❀

to make a thick paste. Massage all over the face and neck. Let this dry for about five to ten minutes. Rinse with warm water and a washcloth to remove. Follow up with a toner of your choice.

Body Exfoliation

BODY EXFOLIATION HELPS TO ease dry skin, prevents ingrown hairs caused by shaving and waxing, and helps the skin on your body to absorb moisturizers. I recommend a body scrub once a week to keep skin feeling soft and refreshed.

Body scrubs are invigorating and very easy to make. They should be applied in the shower. Always apply them before shaving your legs, rather than after, to prevent irritation.

DON'T GET STEAMED

❧

Steaming your face as part of a home facial is unnecessary. Steaming is used in a salon facial to open the pores for the purpose of extracting clogs. If you are inexperienced at this technique, avoid steaming. It can be dangerous and may dehydrate the skin.

Cream of Wheat Body Scrub ND O S: Simply mix ½ cup regular Cream of Wheat (not instant) with 1 egg white and ¼ cup of vegetable oil. Rub all over the arms, legs, and torso. Rinse in the shower. Do not mix this recipe ahead of time, or the cereal will become too soft to be effective. Apply a moisturizer and enjoy your silky skin.

Salt Scrub ND: Mix ½ cup iodized salt or Epsom salts with ½ cup vegetable oil. Scoop up mixture with your fingers and begin rubbing all over your legs, arms, and torso. This application should be done in the shower on damp skin, but try not to let the shower wet the area you are rubbing, because the water can dissolve the salt. The longer you rub, the smoother your skin will feel. Rinse in the shower, and then follow up with shower wash. This mixture is a little harsh for the face, so avoid working it above the neck. Apply a moisturizer after towel drying.

Sugar Scrub $\mathcal{O}$: Mix ½ cup sugar with ½ cup vegetable oil. Scoop up the mixture with your fingers and rub all over your arms, legs, and torso. The longer you rub, the smoother your skin will feel. Shower off, and follow up with a shower wash. This mixture is gentle enough to use on the face, as well as on the body.

Cornmeal Scrub for Very Dry, Rough Skin $\mathcal{D}$: Mix ½ cup cornmeal with 1 egg yolk, ½ of a lemon, and ¼ cup vegetable oil. Rub all over the arms, legs, and torso. Rinse in the shower and follow up with a shower wash. Your skin will feel a lot smoother and you'll feel invigorated. The lemon juice has citric acid, which will help loosen extra dry skin. Apply a heavy moisturizer to the skin while still damp.

Facial Acid Treatments

IN THE BEGINNING OF this book I outlined the new wave of skin care involving fruit acids. Fruit acids help to dissolve the bonds between the already dead skin cells that are about to be sloughed off. Your skin will feel softer and appear more youthful if you aid nature a bit in the sloughing process. I recommend an acid treatment in the form of a mask at least once a week. This should be performed on a day other than scrub day, or you may irritate the skin. People with very dry skin can usually tolerate a scrub and an acid treatment on the same day; just pay attention to your face. You will feel it if you're overdoing it. Signs to look for are redness, stinging, or burning.

My Favorite Acid Treatment—Strawberry Mask $\mathcal{NDO}$: Smash 2 or 3 strawberries into a fine pulp, add 1 teaspoon freshly squeezed lemon juice. Stir and smear all over your face. This should be left on for no more than five minutes and then rinsed with warm water. Follow up with toner and moisturizer.

Tomato Mask $\mathcal{NDOO}$: This is slightly milder. Smash up half of a very ripe tomato or 2 or 3 peeled cherry tomatoes. Smear this all over the face. Do this treatment over the sink or in the shower because it is a little messy. Leave on the face for five minutes, then rinse with warm water. Follow up with toner and moisturizer.

Tomato Paste Mask $\mathcal{ND}\,\mathcal{O}\,\mathcal{S}$: This is easy and convenient if you're out of fresh fruit. Simply open a can of commercially prepared tomato paste and smear all over the face. You can brush it on with a simple paintbrush. Rinse after five minutes with warm water. Follow up with toner and moisturizer.

Lemon Acid Treatment for Elbows and Knees $\mathcal{ND}\,\mathcal{O}\,\mathcal{S}$: This is one of my favorite easy treatments for rough elbows and knees. You may have seen Barbara Streisand use this in the film *Funny Girl.* Slice a fresh lemon in half; rub the exposed fruit over your dry knees and elbows. Pat dry with a towel, but do not rinse. The citric acid will help to speed up skin sloughing. Save the lemon halves in a Ziploc bag in the refrigerator for the next use. You may want to mark the bag.

Specialty Masks

MASKS HAVE HISTORICALLY BEEN used to treat special problems you may have with your particular skin type. Not only do masks have a physical effect on the skin, but they also provide many psychological benefits. I find the application of a 10-minute mask to be soothing, calming, relaxing, and sometimes stimulating. The name of the game here is to take 10 minutes to pamper yourself and your skin. These treatment masks should be applied after freshly cleansing your face and can also be applied after a scrub or an acid treatment.

Banana/Honey Firming Mask for Aging Skin $\mathcal{ND}\,\mathcal{O}\,\mathcal{S}$: Smash up half of a ripe banana and add a teaspoon of honey. Apply a thick coating all over your face and neck. Leave it on until it is completely dry. You'll feel a tightening sensation. Remove with warm water. A washcloth will make it easier. Follow with a toner and moisturizer.

Avocado Mask $\mathcal{O}$: Smash up ½ ripe avocado and smear it all over your face. Even though there is a slight amount of oil in avocados, the

REST, RELAXATION, AND REMOVAL

❧

For clogged pores and blackheads, soak gauze squares in a solution of 1 teaspoon of baking soda and 2 teaspoons of water. Lie down and apply the gauze squares to the nose, cheeks, and chin. Rest and relax for 10 minutes, then remove the pads and rinse the face thoroughly with a warm washcloth. Your pores will be clearer because the baking soda softens hardened skin oils.

pH level of 6.0 is beneficial for oily skin and acne sufferers. Rinse with warm water. Your skin will feel moist, but not oily. Follow with toner and moisturizer.

Acne Rescue Mask *O*: This one is so simple and very effective, especially for teens with active acne and blackheads. Pour a teaspoon of unflavored Milk of Magnesia into a paper cup and apply with a small paintbrush or cotton ball all over the face. Let the mask dry completely. Rinse off with cool water to help close the pores. This may also be applied to back and shoulders to help dry up acne. The active ingredient that controls stomach acid also helps to absorb excess skin oil.

Rescue Mask for Very Dry Skin *D*: This mask is great for flaky skin following too much sun exposure. Smash up ½ ripe banana and mix with 1 tablespoon of mayonnaise. Apply all over the face and neck and leave on for 10 minutes. Rinse with warm water.

Time-Saving Masks

TO SAVE TIME ON your weekly facial treatment at home, I developed mask recipes that have fruit acids in the ingredients. These masks will help soothe and moisturize and deliver an acid treatment for exfoliation.

STRAWBERRY CITRUS MASK *O*

4 STRAWBERRIES SMASHED TO A PULP

1 TEASPOON HONEY

1 TEASPOON FRESH LEMON JUICE

2 TABLESPOONS SOUR CREAM

Whip together and apply to the skin in a thick coating with a paintbrush. Leave on the skin for five to ten minutes and relax. Rinse with warm water and follow with a toner and moisturizer.

This batch will be enough for four applications. It may be stored in a plastic container for up to two weeks. You may freeze it and use it later after defrosting it in your microwave.

ORANGE PAPAYA MASK *ND*

¼ PAPAYA, SMASHED TO A PULP

1 TEASPOON FRESHLY SQUEEZED ORANGE JUICE

1 TEASPOON CANOLA OIL

2 TABLESPOONS SOUR CREAM

Whip all the ingredients together to a smooth consistency. Apply a thick coating to the face with a paintbrush. Leave on the skin for five to ten minutes and relax. Rinse with warm water and follow with a toner and moisturizer.

This batch will be enough for four applications and may be stored in a plastic container in the refrigerator for two weeks. It may also be frozen and used later after defrosting in the microwave.

Quick Tips

For Puffy and Red Eyes: Soak two chamomile tea bags in cold water. Blot them on a towel and apply them to your eyes while lying down for five minutes.

Spoons in the Freezer: Keep metal spoons in your freezer. Place the bowl of the spoon over your eyelid or below the eye on the upper cheek area. Presto! The swelling goes down.

Fading Butter: Blend juice from ½ lemon with 3 to 4 tablespoons of margarine. Brush a thick coating on the back of the hands or anywhere you have age spots. Wipe off in 10 to 20 minutes. The spots will begin to fade over time if you apply the recipe twice a week. Store your Fading Butter in a small plastic tub in the refrigerator and label it.

Lemon Juice Fading Secret: Squeeze a drop of fresh lemon juice on a Q-tip and apply it directly to age spots anywhere, including your face. Let the juice dry. This will help to fade spots over time if you apply it twice a week.

To Attack a Blemish: Grind up an aspirin tablet in a teaspoon and add a drop or two of water to make a paste. Dab a small amount directly on the blemish at night. It will be much less noticeable in the morning.

To Ease Redness from a Blemish: Put a drop of eyedrops that reduce redness on a Q-tip and dab it on the blemish. This will help reduce the redness immediately.

· 7 ·

Cosmetics Counter Combat

"In the factory we sell cosmetics. In the store we sell hope."
CHARLES REVSON, FOUNDER OF REVLON

I NAMED THIS chapter "Cosmetics Counter Combat" for a few reasons. Mainly, to help people recognize that big cosmetics companies launch a huge battle to compete for the dollars women spend on cosmetics. Second, I want to arm women with the right ammunition—knowledge—to fight back when cosmetics industries try to get part of their paychecks.

Spending money on cosmetics is a big lure for most women. The cosmetics shopping habit is really inspired by four things women love to do:

1. Spend money on themselves
2. Buy things that make them look good

3. Indulge in small, sparkling packages, the same way they do jewelry
4. Use cosmetics like arts and crafts—its fun

Women Spending Money

WOMEN OFTEN FEEL THE desire to spend money on themselves. It gives a therapeutic lift to their spirits when they venture out to buy a new cream or a new bag of makeup. Sometimes, women just want to throw away the entire cosmetics bag and start over. One reason is because makeup containers aren't as appealing after they've been tossed about for a few months in a purse. Women love brand-new makeup in clean, bright containers. If they ever feel a need for a pick-me-up, they run out to the store for new eye shadow or blush. Guys do the same thing with tools at the hardware store.

The problem with this "spend to be happy" habit is that cosmetics are outrageously expensive these days. An entire bag of makeup from a major cosmetics company can cost over $200. A simple tube of lipstick at the counter can cost $25. Women would be shocked if they knew that the lipstick cost the manufacturer less than $1. The markup in cosmetics is one of the highest industry margins, higher than for cars, clothing, or technical products. The reason cosmetics companies charge such high prices is because *women will pay them.* As women, we feel the need to spend money even if we think the price is high.

Spending to Look Good

LOOKING GOOD IS IMPORTANT to women. They absorb the model and celebrity images around them every day and aspire to these. For guidance, girls may look to magazine or television commercials. Instantly, solutions are right before them—cosmetics. With this jar of cream and this tube of mascara, women can look just like the model in the ad. By putting a certain tube of mascara beside the face of a model with the world's most amazing eyelashes, an advertiser can get women to believe that mascara will make us look like the model. It's magic. As women, we buy into it because we have a strong desire to look beautiful and glamorous.

Women Like Pretty Packages

BUYING COSMETICS IS A lot like buying jewelry. We love pretty, sparkling gifts. Cosmetics companies spend a tremendous amount of money on making the goods look like gifts. Rushing home from the cosmetics counter with our purchases feels a lot like Christmas morning. Some of the items, especially the pretty compacts, look like little jewelry boxes. When the compacts are new and shiny, fresh out of the package, it's like opening a treasure box full of fancy colors, brushes, and mirrors. The allure is strong.

Using Cosmetics Is Like Arts and Crafts

WHEN WE WERE KIDS, we took great delight in art projects, using color crayons and paint boxes to create our first works of art. As adults, many women don't get the opportunity to be creative in an artistic way. Makeup can be a form of artistic expression. It occupies the hands and gives us a creative outlet. Girls enjoy putting on makeup sometimes just to see what they can create. It doesn't matter if the canvas— your face—is the same every day. Perhaps you share this experience.

Cosmetics Companies Know the Needs of Women

COSMETICS COMPANIES ARE EXPERTS when it comes to knowing the needs of women and meeting those needs. Their knowledge that women will spend a lot of money on cosmetics is one reason that skin-care products and makeup have such a high markup. Women have proved time and time again that they will pay a high price for their favorite brands. There is certainly nothing wrong with that. I mainly want to point out that the amount of money you spend does not necessarily equate with the value of the product. I used to buy the most expensive skin-care line on the market when I was a model. I reasoned that I needed the "best" skin care available because I earned a living with my face. Not until I began my training as an esthetician did I realize that the ingredients in that expensive cream were not much different than those in a brand costing one-third the price. I perceived that the cream was superior because of the packaging and the enthusiasm of the salesperson. I believed her claims that the cream would do so much more because she worked behind a fancy counter and was convincing. The atmosphere at the counter contributed to my thinking at the time.

I encourage women to thoroughly question every purchase at the counter, particularly its price. Don't be afraid to ask, "Why is this product so expensive?"; "What does it contain that warrants the price?" You may feel the need to spend money on yourself; that's okay. The money you spend doesn't have to purchase so little. Start training yourself to look for a good value at the counter. Don't give in to a purchase too quickly.

We all want to look good. Looking attractive makes us all feel better about ourselves. But buying "stuff" doesn't mean we'll look better. My best secret to looking better is knowledge. Knowledge is the key. Knowing how to apply makeup will make the biggest difference in your appearance. The hardest thing to convince women of is that most makeup is very similar. The powders, pigments, pencils, and fluids that come in the jars, bottles, and compacts don't vary to a great degree. Some brands just cost more—a lot more—than others. The higher prices have everything to do with packaging and advertising costs. If we stripped down the compacts and tubes to expose the bare makeup, most of us wouldn't be able to detect a great deal of difference

DON'T BE FOOLED

Beware of cosmetics that contain a trademarked ingredient. Many cosmetics companies use simple ingredients for which they file a trademark name, creating a belief that the ingredient is revolutionary and magic.

in how the product worked. I found this out when I began to assemble my own makeup line. I contacted a handful of private label cosmetics companies to launch my own selection of products. What I discovered was astounding. The most impressive thing I found was how inexpensive makeup was to manufacture. At the wholesale level, a tube of lipstick was a mere dollar or two to purchase. A blush compact with a mirror and a brush was only $2.50. The packaging was simple and didn't include a fancy box, so the raw goods were inexpensive. So why do you have to pay $25 for a blush or $15 for a tube of lipstick? You don't have to, *you choose to.*

Most cosmetics are marked up 500 to 1000 percent. Not only that, makeup and skin-care products at the cosmetics counters *never* go on sale. When was the last time you were in the department store and noticed a 25 percent off sign at the cosmetics counter? It rarely happens. The funny thing is that women notoriously love sales. Yet for some reason, we keep buying cosmetics at full price.

When I found out how big the markup was in cosmetics, I actually got angry. I decided that I would be more discerning about what brands I purchased. I began to use the cosmetics counters to learn how to put on makeup; then I became a better shopper, seeking out the colors I needed at a more reasonable price. I refuse to buy overpriced makeup and skin-care products.

As far as loving the beautiful packaging that makes me feel as if I'm buying jewelry, I quickly grew out of that. Once you realize that your pretty makeup purchases all end up worn out in a few months, the appeal of buying dazzling little containers wears off. I recommend that you focus on what's inside and what it will do for your appearance. Try to look beyond the decorative package and choose the right makeup as if it were a tool. The powders and the creams and how to use them are what you should be interested in.

Cosmetics counters are banking on the artist who is tucked away in all of us. The trend at the counters today is to present makeup that makeup artists use. Makeup counters are set up in a very artistic style, almost as if the salesperson were about to paint a masterpiece. The brushes have gotten bigger, fancier, and, of course, more expensive. A set of makeup brushes, "professional style," can cost over $150. The truth is, you can apply makeup quite well with Q-tips and cotton balls. The fancy tools touch the hearts of our artistic souls. Try looking for other sources for makeup brushes. I rely on brushes from the local arts and crafts store. A set of brushes from the fabric-painting section can serve you very well for a fraction of the cost.

Doing a good job with your own makeup can be simple and easy. It doesn't have to be so complicated. Visit the counter as if you were going to an art lesson. Find out how the makeup is to be applied, but don't be intimidated into making a huge purchase in exchange for the lesson. You can take what you've learned and shop for more reasonable equivalent purchases. For more help and advice on how to put on your makeup, see my suggestions in chapter 8, "De-Mystifying Makeup."

The War Zone

SO, YOU'RE OFF TO a shopping trip at the mall and you feel like cruising the cosmetics counters for a new purchase. You may know ahead of time exactly what you need: a new moisturizer, a new lipstick, and a blush to match it. You don't have a particular brand in mind; you just want to look around. The center of every department store is dedicated to cosmetics and, boy, is it a showplace. The atmosphere in the center of the store is tantalizing to all the senses. A mixture of perfumes and aromas drifts about to tease your nose. Glitz and glamour shout from every square inch of available counter and floor space. It is almost too much to take in. Makeup lights help to create that makeup-artist aura. Photography-style umbrella lights are scattered about to recreate the atmosphere of a model at a photo shoot. The fantasy of "Lights! Camera! Action" is put into play to help connect you with the modeling and celebrity world. The counters are loaded with interesting displays and tester bars. They are powerful magnets, designed to pull you into the world of glamour. (Tester bars at the makeup counter appeal to women just as Nintendos and Playstations at electronics stores appeal to men. We can't keep our hands off them.) Observe the array of colorful shopping bags filled with puffs and puffs of colored tissue. Those perky shopping bags are designed to look like gifts, not purchases. Even if we are making a purchase for ourselves, we feel better about spending money when it is wrapped so attractively. You may feel left out of the loop if you don't leave the counter with a major purchase. You may feel as if all the other women will be gorgeous and you won't, unless you spend money on a bag of cosmetics.

Up on the walls and over the counters hang endless photo collections of supermodels. Here's where cosmetics companies bring out the big guns. This is the biggest force that we have to battle: the image of something most of us feel we can't attain. We see the perfect face, the flawless skin, the bluest and biggest eyes, the longest lashes, the pouty lips, and so on. The draw of the supermodel image is a big one. It starts in our homes as we gaze admiringly at them in magazines and on TV. When we get to the department store, there they are again, conveniently hanging on the wall behind a glass case full of makeup. Our brains naturally associate the gorgeous women in the photos with those goodies in the case. In our minds, we reason that using the products behind that counter will make us look like the models on the wall, or maybe a little bit. You might reject this suggestion, but the tendency to associate the image of the supermodel with the product is common. It is exactly why cosmetics companies hire supermodels to represent and endorse their lines of products. Millions of dollars are negotiated every year to snag the most popular faces for a cosmetics endorsement. It is no different than a basketball star like Michael Jordan promoting Nike products. Celebrities and supermodels help sell merchandise.

Now that you know why you feel compelled to purchase, let's focus on *if* you should purchase. This information may not come as a surprise to you at all. You may feel that the cosmetics you love are worth every penny. Perhaps you don't want to change your shopping habits at all. If this information inspired you to question the lure of the cosmetics counter, here are some additional things to ponder. Be aware of the following strategies cosmetics companies employ to get you to spend.

GIFT WITH PURCHASE

What a great marketing idea the "Gift with Purchase" is. This trend started back in the 1970s and boosted sales in a remarkable way. If you purchased a product costing over a certain amount, you'd receive a free gift. A typical scenario would be for you to make a purchase of $18.50 or more to get a cute little collection of the latest new products, absolutely free. Sometimes the gift items seem like an amazing value, packaged well in striking boxes or cosmetics bags. The makeup or skincare items are usually miniature in size and can be very appealing. Full-sized products are included as well. Nearly always, the gift includes a tote or cosmetics bag with the company logo emblazoned across it. You'll help to advertise for the company, that's part of the clever strategy. One drawback for the consumer is that often, the minimum purchase of $18.50 is a bit disappointing. Usually, it's difficult to find a product priced as little as the minimum purchase. The least expensive product in the line might be much higher. Chances are, you purchase an item you don't really need just to qualify for the free gift. Incidentally, the items in the free gift may not be products you need. They are tempting, I agree. This "free gift" marketing strategy is not truly free if you think about it. To offer these little bonuses, the cosmetics company absorbs the cost by marking up its regular products. The gifts are a hook. Not only does it give the cosmetics company a chance to put a new product in your hands, it causes the purchaser to feel obligated to the brand.

Be aware that participating in a "free gift" program really costs you more money in the long run. If you continue to shop for the free gift bonuses, you will ultimately pay inflated prices for cosmetics.

EXPERTS OR SALESPEOPLE

Salespeople at the cosmetics counter have varying degrees of knowledge and experience. For some reason, department stores do not have to be regulated by the government in order to demonstrate and sell cosmetics as salons do. I've never understood this, but it has been suggested that the cosmetics industry has a powerful lobby to avoid the necessity of licensing cosmetics salespeople. Whatever the case, you should know that salespeople are sometimes hired without any prior experience. No license is required by most states to sell cosmetics in a department store. The cosmetics company that salespeople work for usually delivers the training they receive. The training has everything to do with selling and might not include technical training in how skin functions and what skin needs. This doesn't mean that salespeople behind the counter are uninformed. They might have acquired knowledge in skin care and might appropriately be able to make recommendations. It may be difficult for you, the consumer, to determine whether the advice they give is based on scientific skin-care knowledge or sales training.

In the 1970s, one cosmetics giant launched a new line targeting a younger clientele. The company rocketed into immediate success, based on its clinical name and the presentation of a science and medical background. The salespeople wore white lab coats, giving the impression of integrity, cleanliness, and high-tech scientific breakthroughs in skin care. Instantly, women flocked to that counter for this new revolutionary brand. You could push some little knobs around on a "question and answer" box to identify which products would be scientifically correct for you. I actually bought into that entire presentation and used that brand for several years. It wasn't until I was in esthetician school that I analyzed the products in that line. The cleanser was a bar of soap that I found to be harsh. One of the company's skin toners actually had acetone in it (one could remove nail polish with it). Remarkably, this line still sells well today because consumers want so desperately to believe that it is clinically better for their

PRETTY PACKAGING

❧

When standing at the cosmetics counter evaluating a purchase, picture the item you are buying in a simple plain jar without the glittery surroundings of the department store. Does the product warrant the fancy price? If not, shop for a similar cream with a more modest price tag.

skin. Consider looking beyond the fancy lab coats and smocks and re-alize that these are just a uniform for the salesperson. The uniform does not confirm the salesperson's knowledge or how well the brand will work. You must try to determine on your own what salespeople know, and decide whether their recommendation has any merit.

Snob Appeal

Have you ever walked up to a department store counter, cheerfully looking for help, and happened upon a salesperson who immediately sized you up with her cool gaze? It makes you want to shrink away and back-pedal, doesn't it? I have encountered numerous sales associates who were cordial and friendly. Yet every once in a while I meet one who believes that intimidation is the best approach to winning me over. I find this type of salesperson offensive. Many times these sales-people represent the most expensive line in the store. They seem to wear twice as much makeup as anyone else in the department. It is ap-parent that they *really love makeup* and seem to feel that the rest of us don't get it. When you seek a product recommendation, they may be quick to inform you that their creams are the most expensive. "After all, don't you deserve the best for your skin?" Don't be bullied or in-timidated by this type of salesperson's approach. It is an archaic style of selling and serves no purpose. Women are too smart for that. Simply say, "No, thank you. I'm not looking for the most expensive cream, just the most effective," and walk away. A reliable salesperson should be able to understand the client's needs, even if price range is an issue, and make a suitable suggestion.

Salespeople Are Carefully Selected

Cosmetics companies do a great job of selecting people who look the part. An attractive, well-put-together man or woman may be at the counter to help you. Just remember, what these people look like may not have anything to do with their knowledge. You must still ask ques-tions and insist on good explanations as to why they recommend a product. Sometimes, though, how a salesperson looks can be a guide to that person's makeup style. If a sales associate is wearing too much makeup for your personal taste, she may be heavy-handed when doing your makeup. If you're going for a natural look, which is my suggestion, watch for a makeup artist sporting a more natural, fresh appearance.

Overselling

Talented salespeople can turn a lipstick sale into a five-item sale very quickly. Here's how it works. You ask to try on a new lipstick. The salesperson first puts on a lip primer, explaining that you'll need it to keep the lipstick from running or changing color. Then the salesperson lines your lips with a matching lip liner, saying, "You must use this to define your lips and keep the lipstick from feathering." Now the lipstick is applied with a brush that you need to buy because, of course, a brush is more accurate. Then you need a lipstick sealer to make the lipstick last all day and finally a lip-gloss to keep lips moist or for an evening effect. A super salesperson will also insist that you go home with a vitamin E stick and lip exfoliator to keep your beautiful lips in top condition. Voila! You just spent $100, even though you thought you just needed a lipstick. You may unwillingly buy the whole package because you feel so obligated to the salesperson who spent so much time helping you. Have the courage to stick to the original purchase. Buy only what you will truly use. If a simple lipstick tube is all you need for your lips, so be it. Take a defensive stand against overselling.

There are no requirements that you must follow when it comes to cosmetics.

CUSTOMER BLEND

"Custom Blend" usually means "high priced." Having your makeup custom-blended for your face should not cost any more than regular-priced foundation or powder. The fact that the makeup is blended for you from bulk containers should create a lower price point. Shop carefully for a custom-blended line that serves your pocketbook well.

In other words, you don't have to buy all the possible elements that can fit into a makeup bag. Some women do not need a concealer, just a light foundation. You may be one of the lucky women who can forego the need for powder or eyeliner. Everyone is different. A fresh and natural look can require minimal makeup. Try things out for yourself a little at a time. You, not the salesperson, must be the decision maker.

Negative Selling

Here's my pet peeve when it comes to selling styles at the counter. I cringe at salespeople who point out your faults to get you to buy something. Comments like, "Oh, your skin looks very dehydrated!"; "You're going to need a concealer for your dark circles"; or "How old are you?" Once the problem is identified or pointed out, these salespeople rescue the client with an immediate solution that just happens to be at their fingertips. The client may truly have benefited from the suggestion, but I feel that it is inconsiderate to insult people just to encourage a sale. When I have a guest in my salon seeking advice on makeup, skin, or hair care, I listen and address the problem the client has brought to my attention. I deal only with the client's inquiry. Even if I notice other areas that I could assist in, I tread very carefully to find out if further advice is welcome. This is because a big part of beauty starts with each individual's self-esteem. Why bring attention to something that a client may feel perfectly fine about? It's not always advantageous for clients' well-being to march them down the "fix-it" path until they invite us to. Wounding people's inner confidence will not help boost their outer beauty.

BAR FLY?

❋

Tester bars are very public places. Protect yourself by insisting that the makeup you try on is dispensed with a clean or disposable applicator.

If you encounter salespeople who take it upon themselves to review and critique you uninvited, politely excuse yourself and go to another counter for help.

A Review of Shopping Hints at the Cosmetics Counter

1. Ask for the department manager and find out which lines are the least expensive. Investigate these brands first for the best value.
2. Ask for a thorough demonstration on how to use the product. Be inquisitive about the ingredients in order to justify the price.
3. Look for extra-value products, such as combination palettes of makeup. Try to purchase compacts of makeup that already include the applicators or brushes.
4. Don't get swayed by "Gift with Purchase" bonuses. I view them as "apology gifts" for the prices being so high.
5. Find out what the exchange policy is. Some products are not exchangeable.
6. Look beyond the fancy packaging. The pretty boxes and velvet pouches will probably be thrown away as soon as you get home. The goods you are left with should carry the value.

Alternatives to the Cosmetics Counter

IF YOU LEARN HOW to properly apply makeup and cosmetics, you have conquered the biggest obstacle in beautifying yourself. Shopping for makeup and skin-care products can lead you to less-expensive alternatives. Some of the products in your local drugstore may not come in elaborate packages, but can serve you well. A full-service salon will undoubtedly carry an established makeup and skin-care line. The advantage to shopping at a salon is the licensed technical support you will be offered. The prices in a salon are generally less than those of the cosmetics giants. Salon cosmetics lines are available at a lower price because their manufacturers don't spend as much on advertising as the major companies do. Always insist on product education, and always look for a good value. What you do with your cosmetics purchases will far outweigh where you bought them and how much they cost.

· 8 ·
De-Mystifying Makeup

"There is a great difference between painting a face and not washing it." THOMAS FULLER

MAKEUP WAS ALWAYS a mystery to me while growing up because I never understood what it was really for. I bought lots of makeup through high school and college and dabbled at putting it on, without ever understanding how.

In my twenties I was asked to model for a TV commercial and, by accident, began a career in modeling. Then I began to grasp the power of makeup, how it could totally transform your look. The secret was not in the makeup itself, but in how you used it.

Most women identify makeup as the stuff you smear all over your face as a base. I prefer to call this *foundation*. To me, the term *makeup* encompasses all the cosmetics we use to enhance the features of the face. That's actually the secret to makeup . . . *enhancing* the features. You see, it's not the goal to "paint" your face, but to use "paints" to bring out the best features of your face, to look better . . . naturally. So, no matter what you do with makeup, do it naturally.

Foundation

FOUNDATION IS THE PRODUCT you apply to a clean face to make the skin look better. Foundation comes in many colors, of course, but in many consistencies and formulations as well. If you have normal skin, I recommend using a lightweight liquid foundation to lightly coat and smooth the skin. If you have oily skin, I suggest an oil-free liquid. Dry skin can benefit from a cream-base foundation. No matter what formula you use, the most important thing is to get the shade that's correct for you.

Most people try a foundation on their hands first to see if it's a good match. This won't work well because our hands are typically darker than our faces. The foundation should always be tested on your jaw line. Place a dab on your jaw line, then, and most important, let the sample dry for at least one minute before evaluating. *Foundation will turn a deeper shade after it has oxidized in the air.* If you decide too quickly, you'll go home with a shade that's too dark for your skin and it will look "muddy" on your face.

Your foundation should exactly match your skin at the jaw line; otherwise, it will look like a mask and be detectable. Take the time to get a perfect match. This is essential for a "natural" look.

When applying your foundation, use a cosmetics sponge that you can purchase from any drugstore or salon. The best sponges are latex wedges. They will help you apply the foundation smoothly and evenly. Blend the foundation over your entire face, even lightly over the eyelids, and especially over the jaw line.

Eyebrows

YOU CAN READ MORE about eyebrow grooming in chapter 9, "In Search of the Perfect Brow." The reason I start with eyebrows is because I like to apply makeup from the top of the face and work my way down. This is important because you don't want to rest your hand against the face and disturb the makeup you've already applied. For instance, if you begin by applying lip color and then go to the eyes, you may rest your hand against the fresh lipstick and disturb it. For many women over 30, the eyebrows have been over-tweezed through the years and will require a cosmetics-like brow pencil or brow powder to broaden or fill in the brows. At this time, please go to the next chapter to read up on your brows.

Eyes

THIS IS THE MOST important part of my makeup advice, not only because the eyes play such an important role in your overall look, but because eye shadow is the single most misunderstood step in applying makeup. The purpose of eye shadow should be to reshape the eyes to bring attention to your natural eye color and eye shape. The problem is, women get caught up in the pretty look of the actual colors of eye shadow and choose the wrong "color." It's easy to get lured into picking a shadow at the cosmetics counter that is appealing to look at in the eye shadow compact. We get excited about glittery and sparkling shades of blue, silver, purple, and dazzling palettes. I compare this appeal to seeing a sparkling, glittery evening gown. Personally, I almost always would select a classic black velvet gown. Nonetheless, although sparkling eye shadow is pretty in the case, when placed on the skin, anything with a metallic look will tend to make the skin appear more wrinkled.

I have a rule that if your eye tissue is anything less than velvety smooth, choose a matte finish shadow with no sparkles. Second, dark shadows that are used to contour the eye—that is, to deepen the eye—are best if they reflect no light. So I suggest that you choose a matte. When I select a makeup for someone's face, I'm more concerned with creating "lights" and "darks" than I am with painting her face in pretty or vivid colors. This is the hardest point to make novices understand about makeup. I know that you'll "get it" once you try some of my techniques, especially the eye shadowing.

CONTOURING AND HIGHLIGHTING THE EYES

For learning purposes, let's establish that highlighting means to introduce lighter colors to the face—that is, lighter than your natural skin color—and contouring refers to shading or using tones darker than your skin color.

As a makeup artist, the question I get asked most often is, "What colors of eye shadow should I wear?" Well, I can best illustrate my answer with the following reply: "Have you ever noticed a celebrity or model in a black and white photo looking very beautiful?"

Of course, you have. We see them every day in newspapers and magazines, and they look great. Now in those photos, you don't get an indication of what colors of makeup they are wearing. They look great because of the contours and highlights of their faces. That's all makeup is supposed to do, change and recreate a woman's face to a more perfect form of herself.

The first step to glamorous, natural eyes is to make the eyelid pale in comparison to your skin shade. I recommend a beige or oatmeal shade in a matte finish. Stroke the shadow over your entire eyelid generously until you see that your eyelid is definitely lighter than before. (See figure 1.)

Contouring the Crease

The best shape for eyes is almond, with the corners near the temple turned up slightly. To shape your eyes to simulate the almond shape, start at the outer corner of your eye with a soft medium brown/taupe shadow in a matte finish. It's important to start at the temple side of your eye, because the intensity of the shadow should be stronger here and should fade as you move the color toward the nasal part of the crease. You can feel the soft indentation of the eye socket with a brush

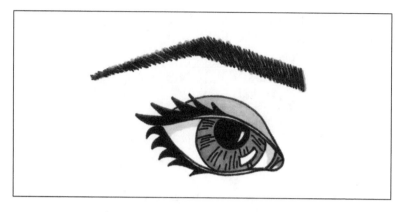

Figure 1. Covering the eyelid for lightening.

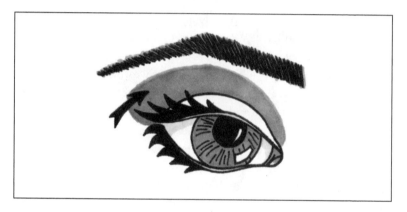

Figure 2. Contouring the crease of the eye with shadow.

as you stroke the shadow in the crease. The natural groove of your eyelid is exactly the contour that you should follow. (See figure 2.)

Deepening the Crease and Lashline

You are now ready to add drama and thickness to the eyelashes. I like to use black eye shadow for this, but you must use it sparingly, for black matte shadow is very potent. Start at the eyelash line at the temple side of the eyelashes. Apply a soft smudgy line to the lashes all the

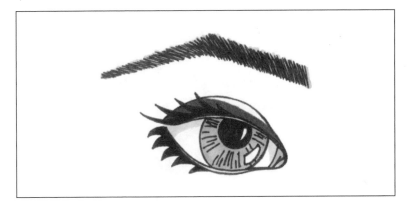

Figure 3. Shading the eyelash line.

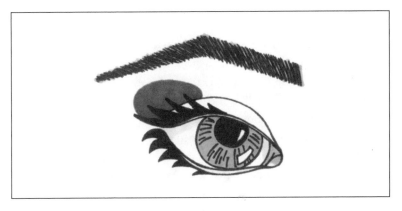

Figure 4. Deepening the outer crease of the eye.

way across, tapering slightly as you near the inside corner of the eye. (See figure 3.)

Next, apply some of the darker color at the outermost corner of the crease area. Keep this new application of the darker shadow in the outer third of the crease area and softly blend with your finger or a clean brush. (See figure 4.)

Last, apply a little bit of the darker shadow on the outer third of the eyelid and blend softly (see figure 5). You will begin to see the development of the glamorous look shown in magazines every day.

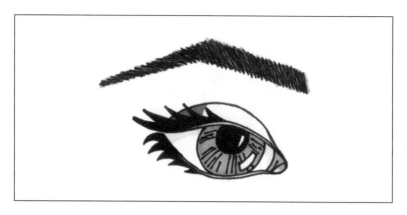

Figure 5. Deepening the outer eyelid.

Eyeliner

The biggest mistake I see women make with eye makeup is that they underplay the eye shadow and use too much eyeliner to try to bring out their eyes. When you encircle the entire eye with a bold black or brown line, you will actually close in the eye, or diminish the size. I use eyeliner to thicken the look of eyelashes, rather than to circle the eye. Therefore, the rule of thumb here is to apply eyeliner wherever there are eyelashes, in proportion to the amount of lashes. There should be a broad line at the outer corner of the eye where lashes are longer and thicker, and the eyeliner should taper toward the inner corner where the lashes become shorter. Never stop halfway across the eye. This is a suggestion I hear a lot from cosmetics counter makeup artists, but I never recommend it because it makes no sense. The liner should cease when the lashes cease. This principle applies to the top and bottom lashes. I recommend an eyeliner pencil in a brown shade for blondes and redheads, as well as light brunettes, and a black shade for dark brunettes and black-haired women. I prefer to use cake eyeliner for the top lashes to create a stronger, cleaner line, but cake eyeliner and a brush require a little more practice to use correctly. Practice painting an arch on your wrist several times before you try it on your eyelid. Pencil eyeliner works well along the lower lashes.

Lashes and Mascara

Many people believe that you should use waterproof mascara to keep
lashes from smudging under your eye during the day. I recommend
mascara you can rinse with water for the following reason: Mascara that
is waterproof is fine for swimming because
it will stay on in water. But remember that
the skin puts out a fine film of oil constantly, and if you use waterproof mascara,
which is oil-based, your mascara will become solvent under your eyes because of
your skin's "oil factor." If you use a mascara you can rinse off, the chances of black
shadowing during the day will be mini-
mized, and your mascara will be easier to
remove at the end of the day.

Mascara Application

Most people start by applying mascara to
the top lashes. Try applying it to the bottoms first. You may find that you'll have
fewer "boo-boos" to the upper eyelids.
When applying the mascara to the bot-

> ### SWEEP YOUR LASHES
>
>
>
> *When applying mascara, make sure to place the wand close to the roots and then stroke to the ends. This will ensure a good lift at the roots to produce that "swept up" effect.*

tom lashes, hold the wand vertically as if it were a candle and the flame
of the candle was going to lick the tips of your eyelashes. This will prevent the wand from brushing across the lower eyelid, which usually
happens if you hold the wand horizontally.

Next, apply it to the top lashes by holding the wand horizontally
and stroking down on the top side of the lashes. This will not only give
the lashes an extra coat of mascara for thickness, but it will take away
the dusty look of the upper lashes by removing the beige shadow you
previously applied to the eyelid. Now apply the mascara to the upper
lashes by stroking up and fanning out the lashes. Keep your gaze
downward while you let the lashes dry.

Blush

AGAIN, REMEMBER THAT WE are applying makeup to the cheeks not just to give the cheeks color, but to create a better shape. The purpose of blush is to lift the cheekbone and give a soft rosy color to the cheeks. I always select a cheek color that is complimentary to the face. A soft neutral rose is a good ticket for almost any face. The blush should be applied in a straight line from the tip of the cheekbone to the hairline at the ear. Don't circle or swirl your brush when applying. Hold your brush at a 45-degree angle to the floor to create a deeper shade at the bottom of the application.

Lips

LIPS SHOULD ALWAYS APPEAR soft and smooth. You may like lip color to be light for daytime and deeper for evening. I tend to agree with that approach. The biggest mistake women make with lips is that they tend to let the lip liner or outline be bolder than the lip color. I like to use lip liner as a guideline and a barrier for lipstick. After you line your lips, apply the lipstick and blend over the lip liner very carefully. If your lip liner shows, it looks as if you have "chocolate milk mouth." It's not attractive.

LIP SHAPE

It's always optimum to have both the upper and lower lip the same size and as full as possible. To shape your lips, use a lip liner and start with the upper lip. Outline the shape of the "V" first (see figure 6).

Next, extend the upper lip line from the "V" to the upper corners. This is very important: Make the upper lip arch out from the "V" to the corners as fully as possible (see figure 7). This trick was taught to me by a German fashion photographer, to give the lip a full line from the profile. Most of us have a "disappearing" lip line at the corners.

Now draw a smooth soft line across your bottom lip, starting from the corners and working your way to the middle. Use small sketches until complete. Fill in your upper lip and bottom lip with lip-

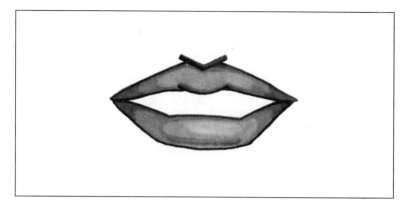

Figure 6. Outlining "V" shape on lips.

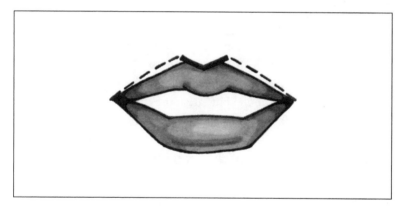

Figure 7. Creating lip arch from "V" shape to corners.

stick straight from the tube or use a brush. Make sure you blend over your lip liner for a natural look.

Powder and Finishing Touches

IT DOESN'T MATTER IF you use a loose powder applied with a big brush or use a compact and a puff. Powder is used to control shine and keep colors from traveling. Apply a light application of powder all over the face and especially under the eyes to prevent mascara from shadowing the lower eyelids. Your makeup is complete. Congratulations!

Touch-Ups

IF WE DIDN'T HAVE blood circulating and oils secreting, or if we didn't move our facial muscles, then makeup would probably last all day. Unfortunately, you will need to touch up your makeup during the day. I recommend a midday reapplication of blush, lipstick, and powder. Your eye makeup should be fine all day unless you have oily eyelids; then you may have to smooth out the crease in your eye shadow.

Evening Makeup

BELIEVE IT OR NOT, I recommend the same palette in the evening as by day, except that I encourage you to apply the colors more strongly. The reason evening makeup should be stronger is that the light sources, such as candlelight, are more dim. Luminous shadows like silvers and golds can be fun to add to your evening look, but remember to add them only after you've created your basic makeup contours.

HOLD YOUR POWDER

Save powdering your face until the makeup application is complete. This will allow you to blend or change your colors before "setting" the makeup with powder.

Ideas and Practice

I GOT MOST OF my makeup lessons in my early days of fashion modeling. I learned my strokes from some of the finest makeup artists in the world. I would stare at the mirror after an assignment and try to duplicate the makeup that had been applied to my face. Fashion magazines are great places to pick up ideas. Find a magazine photo of a model with similar hair and eye coloring to yours. Study the makeup and try to break down visually what the makeup artist did; then try it on yourself. When it comes to cosmetics ads, remember, some ads are trying to get you to buy lots of funky colors and products and may have the model in the photo "rainbow colored." The more expensive cosmetics companies tend to have more classic looks. Try to choose the ad carefully and imitate the look. Practice is the key and can be fun in helping you discover a more glamorous, but natural, you!

· 9 ·
In Search of the Perfect Brows

"If I make a move, like raise my eyebrows, some critic says I'm doing Nicholson. What am I supposed to do, cut off my eyebrows?" CHRISTIAN SLATER

*T*HIS CHAPTER WILL enlighten you on how to correctly shape your eyebrows for the rest of your life. I was one of those girls born with "man" eyebrows, which were a little overpowering as a young teen. Fortunately, I became a woman during the Brooke Shields era and never over-tweezed my brows to try to fit a fashion trend.

In the past few years, the "skinny" brow had a flash-in-the-pan debut, as brow styles often do, and now many women are stuck in the over-tweezed brow rut. What do we do now?

I always caution consumers about going to any old salon for a professional waxing or tweezing because I have witnessed numerous brow mistakes at the hand of licensed makeup artists or estheticians. Unfortunately, licensing doesn't necessarily guarantee good judgment or taste. Go only to professionals who have come highly recommended to you or after you've seen their work.

You can certainly learn to shape your own brows and learn on your own what their correct shape should be. This chapter will provide guidelines for the perfect brow. You don't need to use wax; tweezers will do fine. Oftentimes, waxing is not accurate enough to get a really clean shape, anyway.

Why Are Brows So Important?

WHY, YOU ASK? Have you ever seen a face with very pale or no brows at all? The person looks funny and usually out of balance. Beautiful full brows are the frame of the face, especially the framing of the eyes, which are what we tend to focus on when we speak to someone. If your brows are too thin or too heavy, too round in nature or arched too severely, your entire facial expression changes.

Following are examples of common brow mistakes. Before I teach you how to find the natural guidelines on your face for perfect brows, take a look at your own brows and see if they resemble any of these:

COMMAS

Commas have a thick bulbous beginning and round tails. The brows were tweezed in an arch too quickly and were left too thick at the front. For an example of the comma, see figure 8.

FLAGS

These brows look like flags with a long skinny tail. Too much cleanout was done too severely. For an example of a flag, see figure 9.

CLOWN BROWS

See figure 10 for an example of these. This is so common, reminiscent of the old Bette Davis days. I see these all the time and they require great discipline to grow out. Brows like these will always make you

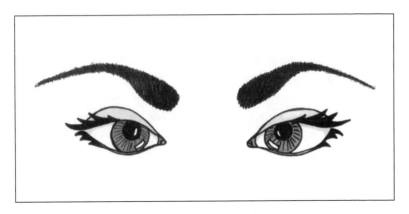

Figure 8. Commas.

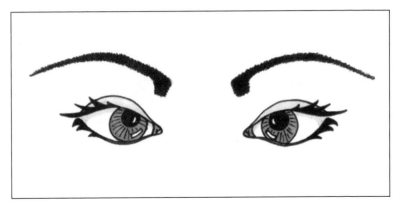

Figure 9. Flags.

look surprised. If you raise the eyebrows in a real expression of surprise, the effect is worse.

Virgin Eyebrows

Before brows are ever tweezed, they may look as bushy as the brows shown in figure 11.

See figure 11 to follow along with the important parts of the brow discussed below. This diagram will point out some key facial guidelines that you need to identify on your own face.

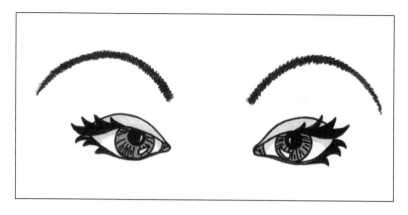

Figure 10. Clown Brows.

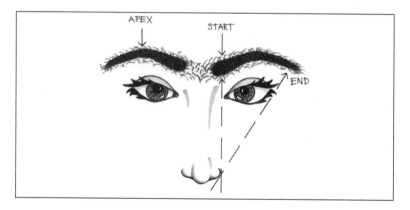

Figure 11. Virgin Eyebrows showing parts of the brow and imaginary lines.

The most important part of the brow is what I call the apex. This is the highest point of the brow or peak of the brow. Most of us have this natural peak, unless you have tweezed or waxed this hair away, making the top of the brow flat. *Never remove hair from the natural apex.* If your apex has already been diminished by inexperienced hands, let the hair there grow back. Leave this area alone until the hair returns.

To find the proper beginning of the eyebrow, imagine a line that could be drawn from the corner of the nostril up to the inside corner of the eye (see figure 11, start). Many times we tweeze out too much hair here and find that our eyebrows have drifted too far apart. If you have tweezed too much hair from in between your brows, let this hair return to match the guideline in the illustration. To find the proper end of the eyebrow, imagine a line that could be drawn from the corner of the nostril to the outer corner of the eye (see figure 11, end). If your brow doesn't extend this far, let the hair return in this area.

The last important guideline is the position where the brow begins to thin out or taper. This point is directly below the natural apex. This point is consistent in most faces naturally, but is often a mystery to women. The misplacement of this point is why so many women end up with funny-looking brows. *Notice that the apex naturally lies directly above the point where the iris or the colored part of your eye meets the white part on the outer side of the iris.* Most women thin out their eyebrows too close to the nose, which will diminish the natural "lift" of the eyebrow. This principle becomes evident in the next drawing.

To the lift the entire eye area, thus making eyes appear more open and alert, the brow should start to thin just under the apex.

Never Say "Arch"

An arch is a curved span between two columns or posts. It is an architectural term, and I never use it when referring to brows because I believe brows look better when they have a straighter, more angular line to them. If you follow my guidelines for a more angular brow, you will see a softer curve develop because the brow itself lies on the curve of your forehead. If your tweezing develops the curve, your brows will end up looking too rounded, or "arched," and the look on your face will one of surprise instead of that alluring, glamorous tilt that we admire on models.

Keep It Straight

When developing the line of your brows, keep the line straight and try not to tweeze out a curve. When you tweeze, use the straight line of the top of the brow as your guideline for the bottom of the brow (see figure 12).

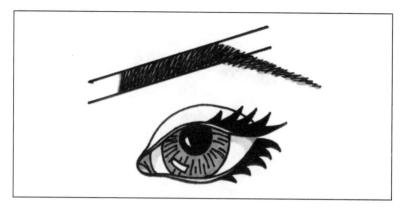

Figure 12. Guidelines to use when tweezing.

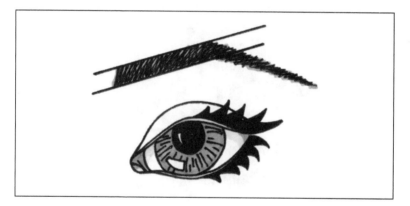

Figure 13. Thinner brow, using the guidelines.

The two lines that are drawn in figure 12 are parallel. This shows that the thickness of the brow at the beginning should remain the same until you get to the apex, then start to taper and thin out. This seems to be the hardest concept for the beginner to grasp. You may decide to have a thinner eyebrow than shown in the illustration. Whatever thickness you decide on, keep the thickness consistent until you reach the apex (see figure 13 and figure 14).

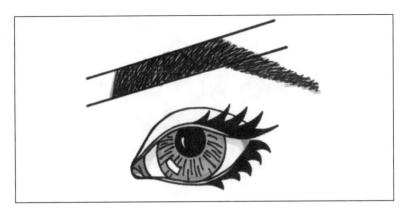

Figure 14. Thicker brow, using the guidelines.

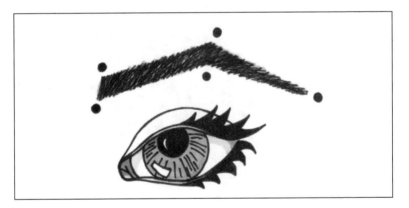

Figure 15. Dot placement for tweezing guidelines.

Practicing Guidelines on Your Face

YOU MAY USE A fine-line red lip liner to place some dots on your brow line so that you can work with the guidelines (see figure 15). After you've placed the dots, take a look at where your brows are deficient or where you need to tweeze. In the beginning, I always recommend that you place these guide "dots" on your face before you tweeze to make sure that you see your guidelines correctly.

Need to Grow

NINE TIMES OUT OF 10, if you are over 25, you will probably have to let much of your brows grow in. I realize that this takes a lot of discipline. None of us want to walk around with new sprouts screwing up our look. It's difficult to be patient and leave the brows alone to return to a more natural shape. If you don't do it when you are relatively young, chances are they may be permanently gone. Don't be surprised if it takes a year for missing brows to fully recover. They will come back, to a certain degree.

HELP IN THE MEANTIME

You can effectively use a brow cosmetic to fill in and define brows to deal with the grow-in process or if you are sure that your brows will not return. I don't recommend brow pencils because they don't look as natural as the new type of brow powders. A brow powder that exactly matches your natural brow shade can look fantastic. I have seen women with absolutely no eyebrows fool everyone with a powder application. Practice using a brow cosmetic until you can make it look believable. It is an important step to your overall look. Don't forget to place your red dots first before beginning to practice. You'll get it in time, and it will be worth it.

MIRROR, MIRROR

❧

To check for shape consistency, lift your chin up and look down toward your mirror. From this different angle, it will be easy to see if your brows are evenly shaped on both sides.

TWEEZING IS A PAIN

Yes, the first time you tweeze your brows, you may vow never to do it again. It may sting, but it will be less painful each time you do it. Pulling the outer side of the brow while you tweeze will help diminish the pain a little. Also, tweezing quickly will feel better than doing it slowly. If tweezing is really painful, try pulling just a few hairs each day until you get the look you want. Once your shape is complete, keep up with it every few days so you won't have to have a big, painful session.

TRIMMING

Bushy eyebrows need to be trimmed, believe it or not, in order to have a clean precise line. So many women don't realize this, and they try to minimize the bushiness with over-tweezing, ruining the shape. To properly trim the eyebrows, brush them up with a brow brush or a small toothbrush. Use a little hair gel on them to hold them in place. Trim them with a small pair of scissors, being very careful working around your eyes. Just trim off the tips, and then check before trimming some more.

Men's Brows

I OFTEN HAVE WIVES dragging in their husbands for a waxing of the brows. Men don't realize how put off we girls get with big, bushy, unruly brows. Some men have an eyebrow that goes across the entire face, commonly called a "uni-brow" or "mono-brow." This look is not only unattractive, it's a huge "no-no" for men in sales or in the public eye. Trimming the brows will improve any man's appearance and so will

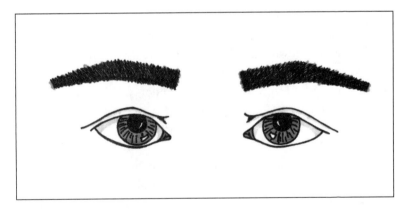

Figure 16. A perfect balance for men's brows.

tweezing the expanse of hair between the brows. Some men who have exceptionally heavy brows can benefit by carefully tweezing a few hairs that lie far below the brow line. See figure 16 for an example of good balance for a man's eyebrows.

Pick a Picture

WHEN DETERMINING WHAT SHAPE of brows are best for you, give yourself a good mental image of what shape you'd like. Look in a fashion magazine and select three photos of models whose brows you like. Study them carefully before you start to tweeze. See the imaginary guidelines on the model's face and then transfer the guidelines mentally to your own face. You should have a better method now of how to approach your own brows. Remember, the brows are the frame of the face.

SHOP FOR BROWS

Keep a collection of magazine tear-out sheets featuring eyebrow styles you like. Having a visual image at hand will prevent you from over-tweezing your brows.

· 10 ·

Mastering Your Own Hair

"To Crystal, hair was the most important thing on earth. She would never get married because you couldn't wear curlers to bed." EDNA O'BRIEN

ISN'T IT AMAZING how the fibers growing from our head can have such an impact on the way we look and feel? When our hair looks good, we feel terrific. On the other hand, if we feel uncomfortable about the style or the lack of styling to our hair, it's not unusual to experience a mood change. The phrase "Bad Hair Day" is a reality with a lot of us now and again. More than anything else, others notice how we wear our hair. We may even feel sensitive to what others think about our hairstyle.

When I started hairstyling professionally, I became acutely aware of how sensitive clients were to their hair and style. For many people, hair is a big part of self-esteem and security. It seems to matter more than makeup, skin care, or even body weight. Men, as well as women, put great importance on their hairstyle. Knowing how critical a hairstyle can be to people gave me a strong desire to be the kind of hairstylist who solved people's hair problems. Not only did I want to design great-looking styles, I wanted to teach my clients how to handle their new hairstyles on their own. I believe that clients should look good every day, not just the day they leave the salon. It is to a hairstylist's credit if her customers receive compliments every day on their hair.

With this principle in mind, I style hair in the salon using a simple, step-by-step process, teaching as I progress through the procedure. I make certain that the client watches and understands what I do and why. One thing that some stylists don't realize is that we're able to style the hair very easily because we are standing above the client's head. Can you imagine trying to style a client's hair sitting behind the client at the same level? I've tried this before, to put myself in the client's shoes. Blow-drying the hair is almost impossible. When customers leave the salon and try to style the haircut I gave them on their own, they need to know how to do it using their own arms. They won't have a set of arms that can magically reach over their head with ease, like the hairstylist's. When you're at home, trying to re-create a hairstylist's magic, remember that the hairstylist did it with the advantage of standing over you. Knowing this clarifies why it is easier for someone else to style your hair than it is for you. You will be just as proficient at achieving the style with a little practice. Make sure that you receive a step-by-step guide to styling the new haircut. Competent stylists should be happy to take the time to teach you, even if they are running behind in their schedule.

My techniques will aid you in mastering hair the same way a hairstylist does. Those of us in the hairstyling world are not geniuses, we're just experienced. By the time we begin cutting and styling hair in a real salon, we've handled hundreds of heads of hair. We make it look easy. You can take comfort in the fact that with a little practice, you'll be more competent and confident with your own hair.

Hair Types

HAIR IS LIKE YARN; it comes in different colors, textures, and weights. Sometimes hair changes during the course of your lifetime. You may have started out with curly hair as a youth and found that it got straighter as an adult, or vice versa. Accept what kind of hair you have and try to work with it when choosing a style. Going "against the grain" often leads to damaged hair and unhappiness. For instance, you may choose to chemically straighten your very curly hair to fit today's smoother hairstyles. Next, you decide to highlight your hair for the streaky, blond look. Those two chemical actions together may severely damage your hair, leaving it unable to do anything. My best advice for hair that is naturally beautiful is to stay close to what you were born with. Slight variations in color or texture are fine in the hands of a good stylist. I will teach you how to safely change the texture of your own hair with some styling techniques and products. If you have curly hair, always seek out celebrities with a similar hair and observe the styles they wear. I suggest the same for people with straight hair. Sometimes we feel better if we can relate to an actress, model, or public figure. Identifying with someone who has the same physical attributes as you may be a better approach than fighting what you were born with.

Here's an explanation of terms I will use to describe hair and hair types:

1. *Straight:* Hair that does not have a wave or curl pattern
2. *Wavy:* Hair that has a little bend or wave to it, not curly, but not completely straight
3. *Curly:* Hair that has a definite curl pattern
4. *Fine:* Hair with strands that are smaller than normal in diameter
5. *Medium:* Hair that is normal in diameter
6. *Coarse:* Hair that is larger than normal in diameter
7. *Wiry:* Hair that is coarse and somewhat unruly, such as gray hair

8. ***Thin:*** Hair that is less dense than normal
9. ***Thick:*** Hair that has a lot of density

You should be able to use three of these terms to describe your hair type. For example, my hair is wavy, thin, and fine. That translates to a head of hair that has a slight wave pattern. I have fewer strands than most people do and my hair shafts are very small in diameter. To make my hair look good, I have to style it with techniques to build volume and thickness. My hair will look as if it has some body because it's wavy. Wavy hair is also easy to curl and holds a style fairly well. My hair has the advantage of wave, even though it has the disadvantage of being fine and less dense than most people's hair. Once you determine the type of hair you have, you will be able to learn how to handle it properly.

Choosing Your Hairstyle

CHOOSING A STYLE FOR your hair is a big decision. Styles change a lot from year to year, making the decisions even tougher. In chapter 3, "Landing the Look," I touched on using fashion magazines to guide you when you shop for clothes. Fashion magazines can also be helpful in determining the trends in hairstyles. When looking through magazines, stick with the fashion editorials for clues on what's "in" for hair. Remember to filter out the wild and outrageous trends that are spliced in with the more classic and wearable styles. Editorials can run the gambit of reasonable to ridiculous. Pick out the obvious details, like straight or curly, long or short, smooth or textured, tailored or shaggy. Tear out some pictures of hairstyles you like and put them in a folder. Have a few options selected. This is important, because certain styles may not be realistic for your hair type. It's a good idea to present some alternatives to a hairstylist, in case your hair limits the options.

My source for "style shopping" is the hair magazines found in the magazine section of the grocery or bookstore. More than a dozen publications come out monthly, devoted to haircuts and styles. Many of these magazines feature celebrities who will be familiar to you from the entertainment world. I prefer the magazines to fancy hairstyling books found in salons, mainly because the magazines are fresh and current. Hairstyling books tend to have styles that feature the art and talent of a certain hairstylist. The styles presented are often avant-garde and interesting, but not natural or wearable. Purchasing a magazine before you go to a salon for a new style will give you a communication tool. Pictures are visual aids and will allow you to show the stylist what you're thinking about for your new style.

I've heard that some stylists reject being shown a picture because they want to choose which style will be best for the client. Unless your stylist knows you very well, or vice versa, insist that you have a hand in directing that person toward a style that appeals to you.

Once you are in a hairstylist's chair, show the stylist the folder or magazine with the styles that caught your eye. Ask whether your hair type would lend itself to any of those styles. Your hairstylist should be able to analyze whether or not the styles you selected are achievable with your hair type, which should help you narrow down the choices instantly. Thick heads of hair lend themselves better to some styles than others. Certain styles you select may be difficult to achieve with your head of hair.

When I counsel clients on a new style, I need to know what their schedules are like. If they plan to spend enough time on styling their hair, then I feel comfortable choosing a more complex style. If they tell me they have a hectic schedule or are rushed for time, I'll choose a style that's easier to handle. Clients should ask how much styling time is necessary to work with a new haircut. Not considering the time factor may make them frustrated when styling their fresh, new look.

After a decision has been reached and the cut is complete, pay close attention to what the stylist does to dry and finish the style. Ask questions and follow the styling technique, step-by-step. You need to know which styling products to use, what kind of brush or comb you'll need, and what direction to blow-dry your hair. Don't leave the salon until you feel confident that you can handle it at home. You can't be married to your hairstylist! This individual won't come to your house every other day and blow-dry your hair for you.

Shampooing and Conditioning

KEEPING YOUR HAIR CLEAN and healthy is the first step in managing your hair. Most of us shower daily, and for many people, this includes a daily shampoo of the hair. There is nothing wrong with cleansing the hair and scalp every day. The only drawback is that it leads to having to style your hair every day. Time, or lack of it, seems to be the subject of everyone's conversation when it comes to hair. A big time-saver for busy people is not to have to style their hair every day. Unless your hair is very oily, you shouldn't have to shampoo daily. After working with hair for so many years, I learned that most heads of hair stay clean for two to three days. Try to change your shampoo routine so that you cleanse the hair every other or every third day. Styling your hair will be more enjoyable if you don't have to tackle it so often.

The frequency that you apply a conditioner will vary, depending on the condition of your hair. Hair in a virgin state (meaning that the hair has been unchanged by chemicals) may not even need a conditioner. If your wet hair is easy to comb without tangling, skip a conditioner. Normal or damaged hair that tangles easily requires a conditioning after every shampoo. Two types of conditioners work well. The first is a rinse-out conditioner that you use in the shower after shampooing. It should make hair easier to comb out, but will not leave a heavy buildup on the hair. The second, newer option is a leave-in conditioner. After you shampoo and towel-dry the hair massage the conditioner into the hair and leave it in. I love leave-in conditioners, especially for hair that is dry or damaged. The hair will respond nicely to blow-drying and hot curling irons. Ask your hairstylist to select an appropriate conditioner for your hair. It is an important step to maintaining a successful style. It will keep your hair looking healthy and shiny.

Towel-Drying

During the rest of this chapter, I use the phrase *towel-dried hair.* I really mean "towel-squeezed hair." Rubbing and drying the hair vigorously with a towel roughs up and damages the cuticle of the hair. A better habit is to squeeze the excess moisture out of the hair to prepare it for styling.

All the Right Tools

Having the right tools makes all the difference in the world when it comes to successful hair styling. Think about all the bottles and hardware that hairstylists keep at their hair stations. There are at least 10 bottles of "goop" at my station and three drawers full of combs, brushes, irons, and dryers. My big collection of tools is to accommodate many different types of hair. You need only the tools that are appropriate for your hair. As a general rule of thumb, most styles can be achieved with a brush and a blow dryer, a styling product, and a finishing product. Blow-drying can require two-handed coordination and is difficult for some people. Alternatives to blow-drying include using a curling iron, flat iron, rollers, and hot brushes. You may or may not know what all these tools are, so this quick overview will familiarize you with what's on the market:

Hardware

1. ***Blow Dryer:*** A handheld, gun-style dryer, designed to dry hair quickly with fingers or a brush.
2. ***Hot Brush:*** A handheld, wand-style blow dryer with a round brush attached. Hot brushes make it easier to dry and brush with one hand. Many clients find this much easier to use than a regular blow dryer. It is especially well suited for making curly hair smooth and straight. Look for one that has short bristles in the brush, to prevent hair from tangling.
3. ***Curling Iron:*** A handheld round metal wand that heats up to curl or smooth the hair. Choose a clip iron, rather than the

Marcel iron that hairstylists use. It will be easier to handle.
Curling irons come in several diameters. To smooth and
straighten hair, choose a larger one that measures 1½ inches.
For making curls, choose a smaller one from ⅜ to ¾ of an inch.

4. *Flat Iron:* A handheld iron with a paddle head, used to iron
out hair smooth and flat. They are great for making curly or
kinky hair straight. Try to find one that has a temperature
control. Flat irons are exceptionally hot, so avoid using them
every day.

5. *Hot Rollers:* Rollers that heat up in a dry heat or steam unit.
They come in many sizes. Choose a set that has medium to
large rollers. Rollers can be very hot and should not be left in
the hair a long time. The hair will become very dry from using hot rollers daily.

6. *Regular Rollers:* Rollers come in many sizes. Smooth rollers
are made of plastic and require clippies to keep in place. I
prefer self-adhering rollers, which are plastic rollers with a
Velcro-type coating. They stay in place without clips and are
very easy to use. For smooth and straight styles, select large
rollers. For curly styles, use smaller rollers.

7. *Yoyettes:* Metal or plastic clips that are similar to clippies but
longer in length. These are very important tools to divide
your hair into sections for blow-drying or using hot styling
tools. You may need as many as 10, depending on how much
hair you have.

8. *Clamp Clips:* Plastic "jaw"-style clips that can also be used to
divide the hair into sections. You may need four to eight of
them, depending on how thick your hair is.

9. *Round Metal Brush:* A round metal-based brush with plastic
bristles, used to shape the hair while blow-drying. These
brushes are ideal and versatile. They are available in many
sizes, from ½ inch up to 2 inches in diameter. Your stylist
should recommend the size that will work best with your cut.

10. *Round Natural Boar Bristle Brush:* Ideal for straightening curly
hair. Ask your stylist for the size that's suitable for your style.

Liquid Styling Tools

1. ***Mousse:*** Styling foam designed to give a lightweight hold and volume to the hair. Mousse is best suited for fine lightweight hair to give shape, volume, and lift. Apply to towel-dried hair before styling.

2. ***Gel:*** A thick gelatinous substance designed to give a firmer hold to the hair. A good gel should not flake after it dries. Gels are usually used to give hair a wet look and are best suited for men or shorter hairstyles. Some gels are lighter weight and come in spray form. These are good for distributing throughout a thick head of hair or long hair.

3. ***Curl Enhancers:*** A liquid in a spray form that aids the curl pattern in hair. These are beneficial to perk up a perm or curly hair. They should be applied to wet hair to help keep the integrity of the curl.

4. ***Root Lifters:*** A foam or liquid designed to lift the base of the hair off the scalp. These are fairly new on the market and aid tremendously in giving volume and thickness to thin, fine hair. They work so well to give lift, I recommend them over getting a permanent wave. Apply a root-lifting product to towel-dried hair before styling.

5. ***Pomade:*** This comes in many forms, such as foams, waxes, sprays, and creams. It is designed to shine and polish the hair and to give texture and separation. The hardest decision to make is which one is best for your style. Ask your hairstylist to recommend the appropriate formula. Pomade is used on dry hair to finish the style.

6. ***Hairspray:*** A pump-type spritz or aerosol to hold the hairstyle. Hairsprays vary, from light to firm-holding. Just remember that the stronger the hold, usually the more alcohol is used, which can be drying. If you restyle your hair throughout the day, be sure to select a spray that is easy to comb out, so you don't break your hair.

My Secrets for Successful Hairstyling

MY SECRETS ARE DESIGNED to achieve the hairstyle while saving time. If I can save you time, the task will be more enjoyable and you'll be more consistent about styling your hair.

We'll assume that you already have a new haircut and basically know what it should look like. My styling techniques should help once you get home from the salon.

BLOW-DRYING

Select your favorite styling product and work that into towel-dried hair. Comb the product through the hair to remove tangles and distribute the product evenly. Begin blow-drying your hair with your head upside-down. The best way to accomplish this is to stand rather than sit, and bend over slightly at the waist. The idea is to dry the roots while the head is upside down, to give the hair fullness and help create volume. You may lift the hair away from the scalp as you aim the dryer at the root area. Be sure to move the dryer around so that you don't heat up the scalp. Spend enough time in this position to get the hair 80 percent dry. It will make styling the rest of your hair easier.

Once your hair is nearly dry, stand up straight and set your dryer down. Now it's time to section your hair. Using yoyettes or clamp clips, section your hair into several layers. Start with the very top of the head and secure it with a clip. The next layer is the temple section. You may section this part of the hair with two clips, one for each side. The third section

IT'S IN THE ROOTS

The most important time spent on your hair is the time you take to dry the roots. This will produce extra volume and shape. Remember this key phrase: "Slow down to style the crown." Thoroughly drying the roots at the crown will give you a lift in the back on the head where many of us tend to be flat.

includes the hair above the ears and to the back. Secure this with one clip. Now you should be left with a large section of hair hanging down the back. Divide this hair into top and bottom; secure the top half with a clip, leaving the bottom half hanging down. Now you are ready to continue blow-drying with a brush in sections.

Using a brush in one hand and the blow dryer in the other, finish drying the bottom section thoroughly. It should only take three or four passes of the brush and dryer to complete the section. You may choose to blow the hair turning under, flipping up, or just pulling the hair straight.

Set your dryer down and remove the clip from the top half of the back section. Proceed with dryer and brush. Dry this section thoroughly before moving on to removing the clip that holds the next section. Finish drying the hair one section at a time, always from the bottom to the top. By breaking the hair up into smaller sections, you can manage the style much easier by yourself. You won't become frustrated by getting the brush stuck in the hair. Most important, by drying in sections, the hair will take on a better shape and the style will last longer throughout the day. Drying the hair all at once doesn't give it a chance to dry completely. If you quit styling when the hair is still damp, especially at the roots, the style will be incomplete or will "poop out" in about an hour.

Once you've completed the top section, wait about one minute before putting the finishing products in. This will give the hair a chance to cool, which sets the style.

No Static!

To fight static in brushes or combs, spray a light mist of "static guard" or similar antistatic fabric spray. This will help fight static and won't harm your hair or hairstyle.

ALTERNATIVES TO BLOW-DRY STYLING

Blow-dry styling can be awkward for some individuals. If you have trouble operating a dryer and a brush, here are some other methods you can try:

1. ***Hot Brush:*** After drying your hair upside-down until it is 80 percent dry, section your hair with clips, then proceed with a hot brush. You'll still work in sections from the bottom up. Then continue with finishing products.

2. ***Rollers:*** This is my favorite method and the one that I use on my own hair. Blow-dry the hair upside-down to get volume at the roots. Dry the hair completely this way. Stand up and, while the hair is still warm, set the hair with self-adhering rollers. Spray the hair with a lightholding hairspray and wait for about 10 minutes. Take the rollers out gently so that you don't disturb the style, and then continue with finishing products.

3. ***Curling Iron:*** Blow-dry the hair upside-down to achieve volume at the roots. After the hair is completely dry, divide and clip into sections. Work the curling iron through the hair, one section at a time, starting with the bottom and working your way up. For a straight style, simply clamp the iron on the hair section and stroke the iron down the hair to smooth and straighten out the hair. To curl the hair, stroke each section first with the iron, then wind the hair around the iron and hold for only two or three seconds. Avoid the habit of baking the curl in with a hot iron. You will dry the hair out.

4. ***Flat Irons:*** Follow the same procedure as explained in the previous curling iron section. Remember that flat irons are very hot and can dry out the hair. It is better to stroke the hair a few times quickly than to iron the hair very slowly. Using a leave-in conditioner will help to insulate the hair from hot irons.

5. ***Hot Rollers:*** The only drawback to hot rollers is that they get extremely hot and will dry out the hair if used with great frequency. Hot rollers tend to give the hair an old-fashioned look. If you use hot rollers, leave them in for no more than five minutes. Try a new styling technique if you are in a hot roller rut.

DRYING CURLY HAIR

Curly hair is a blessing and a curse, depending on what you wish to do with it. If you have curly hair and want to wear it curly, then the styling game is easy. Straightening curly hair is a different story and requires a little more effort. Hair that is curly will respond better with a little extra conditioning. Try using a conditioner in the shower and a leave-in conditioner in tandem. The beauty of curly hair is that you can go longer between shampoos.

Drying Curly Hair in a Curly Style

You will need a blow dryer with a diffuser and some clippies. A diffuser is an attachment for your blow dryer that breaks up the force of the dryer to avoid blowing the curls around. It really helps keep the curl pattern consistent and prevents frizzing of the hair.

After applying a leave-in conditioner to wet hair, spray a liquid spray-gel all over the hair and comb through with a wide-tooth comb. Using your hands, squeeze and scrunch the hair to form a curl pattern. The next step is a cool trick. It is designed to keep the hair curly up at the root area on top of the head where curls seem to drag out. The reason curls drop or flatten out at the scalp, especially with long hair, is because of gravity. When your hair is wet, the water in the hair tends to travel down the hair, adding weight to the ends. This extra weight pulls downward on the hair and straightens out the curls at the top of the head. To prevent this, you need to take the weight off the curl pattern at the top. Using clippies, clip the hair in small sections at the top of the head, one inch away from the scalp. The idea is to open the clip, place it in the hair, and shove the hair up about a half an inch toward the roots. You may use eight to ten clippies to accomplish this. As the hair dries, the initial curl at the base of the scalp will have a chance of surviving the weight of the wet, heavy hair.

Now proceed with drying the hair, using the diffuser. You may bend over and hold your head upside-down, letting the hair gather in the basket of the diffuser. Push up to further scrunch the curl pattern into the hair. Continue drying until the hair is 80 percent dry. I don't dry curly hair completely in order to limit the amount of frizzing. Don't forget to remove the clippies.

Drying Curly Hair in a Straight Style

You will need to know how to section the hair with yoyettes. Please refer to the section in this chapter that explains the basic blow-drying technique. Before you start, it's important to give the hair the advantage of a product designed to straighten curly hair. Curl tamer is a more specific leave-in conditioner that you can get at a salon. Not only will a curl tamer aid in getting hair straight, it will keep the hair from curling up in humidity. Curl tamers make curly hair feel smoother and less frizzy. Put an abundant amount in wet hair, then section it before you blow dry the hair in the upside-down method. Exceptionally curly hair needs to be straightened while it is still wet. If you try to partially dry it, then straighten it, you may not be as successful in removing the curl. Use a natural boar bristle brush that is round in shape. It will be the most effective in grabbing the hair to pull it straight. Use a brush with short bristles, as round brushes are notorious for getting stuck in the hair.

Proceed to straighten the hair one section at a time, starting from the bottom and working your way up to the top. Straightening a curly head of hair requires patience. Once your hair is completely straight and dry, you may choose to sleek it a bit more with a curling or flat iron. Be sure to re-section the hair in clips before you go back through it with the iron. Because the straightening process is time-consuming, try to go two to three days between shampoos.

FINISHING YOUR STYLE

The biggest secret to ensure that you look salon-finished after styling your own hair is what I call the "Last Five Minutes" technique. Hairstylists deliver most of their magic in the last five minutes of styling. By the time you get finished with your blow-drying procedure, you may be tired of working with your hair. The secret to great-looking hair is to be patient for five more minutes to finish the look. This is when you should use a finishing product like pomade to give the hair an extra bit of texture and shine. Pomade helps to separate and detail the hair, giving more

SCRIMP & SPRAY

Don't spray hairspray in a cloud all over your head. It's unhealthy for your lungs and unnecessary. I recommend a dash of spray just where you need it for hold. Hair should be free to move a little bit; otherwise, you will look old-fashioned, with the "helmet head" look.

dimension and shape. At this point use your fingers more than a comb or a brush. Have a picture from the magazine handy as a visual aid. Don't give up until you like the way it looks. Use a hairspray to hold the finished look.

Practice makes perfect, and you'll get better each time you patiently work with your hair. If you're not getting the hang of it, call your stylist and ask if you can come in for some further styling hints. A good stylist will be more than happy to help you.

More Helpful Hints

1. Get regular hair trims or cuts even if you are trying to grow your hair long. Not trimming the hair in an effort to save length will cause ragged ends to break further.

2. For healthy hair and hair growth, eat a well-balanced diet. Foods high in folic acid are beneficial for healthy hair growth.

3. Beware of using rubber bands to tie back hair, as they tend to cause breakage. Use coated or fabric bands to prevent breakage. Remove them slowly and carefully.

4. Never speed through the combing-out process, especially when your hair is wet. Damage and breakage to the hair are self-inflicted when we are in a hurry. Hair in a wet state is more fragile than you think. Use a conditioner and detanglers to aid in combing the hair. Use a wide-tooth comb first, then a small-tooth comb or brush.

5. To disguise split ends, use a dab of petroleum jelly on the fingers and lightly stroke on dry hair ends. Get regular trims to prevent dead ends.

6. If you have a dry or flaky scalp, brush the hair and scalp before shampooing with a natural boar bristle brush. Many times a dry scalp simply needs to be exfoliated with a good brushing.

7. To make hair shiny, rinse in ice-cold water. This can be somewhat uncomfortable, but you can rinse the hair, not the scalp. The cold water closes down the cuticle layer of the hair, leaving it smooth and shiny.

8. For oily hair or limp hair, avoid conditioning at the scalp. Conditioner can be applied just to the ends and mid-shaft.

9. For a natural detangler, rinse hair after shampooing with a tablespoon of apple cider vinegar mixed with a glass of warm water. Comb through the hair, then rinse with cool water.

DON'T BE FOOLED

Home hair color is not as easy as manufacturers lead you to think. The hydrogen peroxide in home hair color kits is designed to suit all hair types and can be somewhat harsh. You may be sacrificing the health and integrity of your hair just to save a little money. See a professional hairstylist, or economize by seeking help at your local beauty college, where the work is supervised by a licensed teacher. It's worth it!

TREAT YOUR HAIR TO A SPA REGIME

Give your hair a break from your normal routine by treating yourself to a spa hair treatment. The benefits will be rewarding for your hair's condition and will boost your sense of well-being.

Draw a warm bath while you brush your scalp thoroughly with a natural boar bristle brush. Take your time. Get in the tub, wet your hair, then massage in your favorite moisturizing shampoo. Dip your fingertips into your favorite essential oil and massage into the scalp. Try lavender, chamomile, orange, tea tree, or ylang ylang. Press your fingertips into the scalp and move the scalp around to stimulate circulation. Rinse your hair thoroughly. Apply a deep conditioner and put a plastic shower cap on your head. Relax in the tub and allow 10 minutes for the conditioner to work. Rinse the hair when you are ready to get out. Comb your hair out and allow it to air dry. This relaxing spa treatment for your hair can be a once-a-week or once-a-month experience.

HOMEMADE MOISTURIZING SHAMPOO

1 EGG

½ CUP WATER

½ CUP GENTLE SHAMPOO

1 TEASPOON VEGETABLE OIL

$\mathcal{W}$hip up the egg until it is well beaten. Add the water, shampoo, and oil. Mix together with a whisk and store in a plastic bottle. This luxurious shampoo will leave the hair shiny and more manageable. It will last for two weeks if stored in the refrigerator.

NATURAL HAIR PACKS
FOR DEEP CONDITIONING

Making a deep-conditioner pack for your hair is simple, using ingredients from your kitchen. My favorite is mayonnaise and avocados. My family humorously refers to it as hair guacamole. It works well because the mayonnaise and avocados are rich in oil.

1 AVOCADO (VERY RIPE)

2 TABLESPOONS MAYONNAISE

$\mathcal{B}$lend the ingredients together to make a smooth pudding. Massage it into hair and scalp (while hair is dry) and place a plastic shower cap on the head. You can wrap a warm, moist towel around your head to help with absorption. Simply dampen a towel and microwave it for one minute at a time until steamy. Be sure to test the towel before wrapping your head.

After 10 to 20 minutes, rinse the pack out of the hair with warm water, then shampoo.

——————————————— VARIATION ———————————————

If your hair is oily and you wish to avoid the mayonnaise, try smashing up a very ripe banana and mixing it with the ripe avocado. Follow the same application procedure as outlined previously.

· 11 ·

The Secrets
of Waxing

*"If you do what you've always done,
you'll always get what you've gotten."* ANONYMOUS

WAXING TO REMOVE unwanted hair is a secret Europeans have known for years. We've just
started catching on in the United States. Waxing has
its roots in the ancient Egyptian era, where a mixture
of honey, beeswax, and sugar was spread on the skin
and pulled off to remove unwanted hair. This ancient
method has stood the test of time. The popularity of
waxing to remove hair has spread like wildfire in the
last few years and for many good reasons. This chapter details my secrets for successful waxing techniques. You will be able to make your own sugar wax
and wax your own legs, arms, and so forth. If you
don't wish to try this at home, you'll be better

equipped with knowledge about waxing so that you may choose a salon professional to perform this service.

The Benefits of Waxing

I AM A BIG proponent of waxing over any other method of hair removal. Here are just some of the advantages to waxing:

1. It lasts four to eight weeks
2. The new hair grows in finer and softer after waxing
3. It eliminates daily shaving, nicks, and cuts
4. It diminishes the rate of hair growth over time

When you have your legs, bikini line, or underarms waxed, you won't have to wax that area again for four to eight weeks. Compare that to shaving every other day. Most women don't have time to spend 10 to 20 minutes every other day shaving in the bath or shower. I have met women who claim that they need to shave their legs and underarms daily or their hair will show. Not only is shaving time-consuming; the hair is coarse and sharp as it grows in, often making legs and underarms feel rough.

The old wives' tale that shaving promotes hair growth is not true. Hair grows at the same rate, no matter how many times you shave. The reason you may feel that your hair gets more coarse from shaving is because the roots remain intact and the hair continues to grow stronger and thicker until that hair falls out in its normal replacement cycle. Shaving the hair simply cuts the hair at the surface. The next day after shaving, the hair will peek out just enough above the surface to feel rough. A man has beard stubble on his face at the end of the day; women have leg stubble the next day. The real problem for women is that we have a lot more square inches to shave on our legs than a man has on his face. It's hard to keep up with shaving when we're busy.

The nifty thing about waxing is that it removes the hair below the surface of the skin. It pulls hair out by the roots. The return cycle of hair growth usually takes three to four weeks. Not only will the hair shaft return slowly, it will bud from the root, thus the hair will be finer and softer. The added bonus, which is the best-kept secret about waxing, is that the root will eventually die, which thus makes waxing a permanent hair-removal method. To achieve permanent hair removal, you may have to wax an area of hair for several years, but it is a far superior method to shaving.

In recent years, it was thought that the only method of permanent hair removal method was electrolysis (the application of an electric current to the root of an individual hair to deteriorate the root). I was a believer in electrolysis and even used to employ an electrologist in my salon. The problem with electrolysis is that it's painful; it's time-consuming, because each hair root must be treated one at a time; and it's very costly. An electrologist usually charges a dollar per minute and treats two to four hairs per minute. Permanent removal may require up to a dozen applications to each individual hair. This method makes sense for small amounts of hair, as in the chin or eyebrow area, but it is absolutely unreasonable for larger areas like the forearms and the legs. The areas of the upper lip and the bikini line are so sensitive that I cannot recommend electrolysis in those areas.

Waxing can be a bit painful the first few times you try it, but if it's done correctly, it's very tolerable, even in the bikini area. The speed with which waxing is performed is the secret to painless hair removal. Large areas of hair can be removed with great speed, making waxing a time-saving technique. Compare a full leg wax service, which takes an hour every six weeks, to a 20-minute shaving session every other day. If you shave, you'll be shaving the rest of your life; the hair will never stop growing. If you wax, chances are you will be almost hair-free after 10 years. I've been waxing my legs consistently for seven years and have one-quarter the amount of hair I used to have. The benefits of waxing are really worth it.

The Principles of Waxing

BASICALLY, A WAXING MATERIAL is spread thinly over skin where hair is present. A sheet of muslin cloth or other material is placed over the wax and rubbed lightly. The cloth is removed quickly, picking up the wax and uprooting the hair. The skin will be hair-free until the root regrows and surfaces. Sounds simple? It is. I will teach you in detail how to properly wax yourself. It is not difficult to do on yourself once you know a few of my tricks. After you've learned how, you may be comfortable enough to do it yourself all the time. If you'd rather not try it on your own, but would like to try it at a salon, be sure to continue reading about my waxing secrets. You'll be better equipped to choose a waxing expert in your local area.

It has been my experience that not all salon professionals wax the correct way. My goal in this chapter is to prepare you to find a knowledgeable person to perform this service.

HAIR GROWTH

Before you actually wax your own legs, arms, or upper lip, I'd like you to know a little bit about hair growth. Hair grows everywhere on your body except for the palms of your hands, the soles of your feet, and your lips. The hair on your body has a growth cycle, just as the hair on your head does. It grows from the root, attains length, then sheds and replaces itself. Hairs that are in the middle of their growth cycle will appear above the surface of the skin. Other hairs that are at the beginning of their growth cycle may be just below the surface of the skin. When you spread wax over the skin, it will remove only the hair that is long enough for the wax to "grab." New hair or hair that lies just below the surface will not be affected by the waxing and will continue to grow, surfacing just a few days after the wax service. It is important to understand this and be patient in letting the hair reach a length that is at least one quarter of an inch before waxing. If not, you may be disappointed in skin that does not feel smooth or hair-free.

Many women have come into my salon for a waxing service with hair that is only two days past shaving. Of course, they are disappointed when we turn them away because their hair is not long enough for the wax to grab. The remark I often hear is, "I can't go a week with my hair growing out!" It requires a little tolerance, for sure, but once you've tried it and realized the benefits, you'll find that it's worth it.

A good test to see if your hair is long enough to wax is to take a dull kitchen knife and spread a bit of honey on the area to be waxed. If the hairs will lie down under the sticky layer of honey, the hair is long enough to be waxed.

WHERE TO GET WAXING MATERIALS

I'm sure you've seen the flood of infomercials in recent years for home waxing kits. You can order basic wax and waxing supplies from television offers or at your local beauty supply shop. I have even seen small waxing kits at the corner drugstore. Most of these commercially prepared products are absolutely fine, but a lot of what you get in the kit is absolutely unnecessary and a waste of money. Unnecessary items are the cleanser to clean the skin prior to waxing and the solvent to remove the residue after waxing. I don't recommend pre-cleansing the skin because this process will remove the protective layer of skin oils. If the skin is pre-cleansed, the wax will stick to the skin and make removing the wax more difficult and painful.

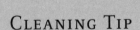

CLEANING TIP

Clean up spills with a wet hand towel that you microwaved for one minute. Clean-up is easy if you use just water and a towel.

The ingredients in the wax mixture may contain lots of different things, some of which are good and others that can irritate the skin. Most products that call themselves "wax" have very little wax in them at all. The most common ingredient in hair removal wax is tree resin. Other things may be added, like beeswax and sugar, but most commercial formulas I've tried are predominately resin materials. Resin waxes can cause sensitive reactions in a small number of people. The other drawback is that they leave a sticky residue on the skin that has to be removed with a solvent. The solvent, of course, is one of the added things they try to sell you with the waxing kit. The solvents that are strong enough to dissolve resins are usually somewhat harsh on certain people's skin. If you use a commercial wax that is resin-based and leaves a residue, I recommend that you rub some good old vegetable oil over the waxed area and remove it with a warm, wet towel. You'll safely remove the residue without causing irritation.

The safest type of wax is made from sugar. Many new wax products made mostly from sugar are out on the market now. *Sugaring* is the new buzzword in salons. Sugar waxes are not as sticky and have been known to be slightly less thorough than resin waxes, but they still do a great job with a lot less skin irritation. The big plus with using a sugar wax is that the sticky residue is removed with water. The cleanup is easy.

Make Your Own Wax

Making your own wax is easy and very inexpensive. Before you try out this homemade recipe, I would strongly suggest that you go to a salon and get a professional waxing service. It is really important that you experience what waxing feels like so that you will be familiar with the procedure. Once you've watched the service done, you'll get the hang of it very fast. I wouldn't want you to make up a big batch of homemade wax and not know what to do with it.

Homemade Sugar Wax

1 CUP WATER

2 CUPS SUGAR

2 TABLESPOONS FRESH LEMON JUICE

Combine the ingredients in a saucepan and bring to a boil. Keep heating the sugar mixture on high, watching it constantly. While it is boiling, bring a second saucepan of water to a boil and have it standing by. The sugar mixture needs to boil until it starts to turn a slightly deeper color. The secret is to cook the sugar just enough to get sticky, but not so much that it gets too firm when cool. It will be ready when the color of the mixture is about the color of ginger ale, just starting to turn golden. It will also be ready when the mixture keeps bubbling for a few seconds in a spoon. To test it, use a big metal spoon or a metal ice cream scoop. Scoop up a spoonful of the mixture and see if it bubbles in the spoon for at least two seconds. If it does, it's ready. Remove the wax from the heat and add 1 tablespoon of boiling water from your second pan. Stir thoroughly and allow mixture to cool slightly. You will want to store your wax in a plastic container with a lid, such as a Tupperware container. Transfer the wax to the plastic container when it is still fairly thin. Add water to the saucepan and bring the water to a boil to help clean the pan.

You must let the wax cool completely before reheating it for use. *Do not try the wax as it is cooling! It will be very warm and unsafe to use.* In order to use your homemade sugar wax, you will need to heat it slightly in the microwave. Microwave it with the lid off for one minute at a time, until it is the consistency of honey. It should only take two to three minutes.

Other Materials Needed for Waxing
✦ Corn starch
✦ Cotton muslin strips, a cotton sheet cut up into strips, or strips cut out of a brown paper bag*
✦ Wooden Popsicle sticks, or a smooth butter knife (no serrations)
✦ Two old, washable towels

For teaching purposes, let's assume you are going to wax your lower legs, from the knees down. I will take you through this procedure to familiarize you with the basic waxing method. After learning or visualizing this technique, you can apply the principles to other areas of the body. I will also map out my secrets to waxing other areas of the body immediately following this leg procedure.

Waxing is a little messy so should probably perform the procedure on some floor space, such as the bathroom floor. Put 2 to 3 tablespoons cornstarch in a bowl and place it nearby. This will be used to pre-powder the skin and to dip your fingertips in to keep the fingers

---

*I like paper bag strips because they are always handy and inexpensive.

from getting sticky during the waxing procedure. Have your cotton strips or paper bag strips (pick-up strips) and Popsicle sticks or butter knife (applicators) beside you on one of the towels.

Bring a small saucepan of water to a boil, then remove from heat and let it stand for five minutes. This will serve as a water bath to keep your wax warm and liquid. Microwave your homemade sugar wax on high for one minute at a time. It usually takes two to three minutes to get the right consistency. The sugar wax should be the consistency of honey. If it is thinner than that, it's probably too hot and will need to cool down for a few minutes. To safely test the temperature of the wax, dip your applicator into the wax and quickly tap the applicator on the back of your hand. It should feel very warm but not hot. Place the wax in the water bath. You are ready to begin.

Place the towels on the floor and sit down on them with your feet out in front of you, as if you are sunbathing. Make sure that you have all of your materials on the side of your body of your working hand. Apply a liberal coating of cornstarch to both of your legs from the knees down. Your legs should look very white. The cornstarch will keep the wax from sticking to the skin. Waxing is much more tolerable when the skin is powdered. This is an important step in waxing that even some professionals don't know. Some salons cleanse the skin with an antiseptic solution prior to waxing. This is a big mistake, as I mentioned earlier, because the skin is stripped of its protective oils and thus the wax removes skin cells, causing wax abrasions. Powdering the skin with cornstarch will protect the skin from this invasive exfoliation.

Next, coat both of your hands with cornstarch. Pretend as if you're rubbing the cornstarch into your hands, like lotion. Now you're ready to apply the wax.

Wax should be stroked onto the skin *in the direction of the hair growth.* For leg hair, stroke down the legs from the knees to the ankles. The hair will be pulled off in the opposite direction. First you must learn to apply a thin, not a thick, coat of wax. To do this, try to think about applying butter to toast as if you want as little butter on the toast as possible. The technique will be a little like scraping down the leg. It sounds as if this would hurt, but it doesn't. Just remember, as you apply the wax, it will work better if you apply a very thin coat. Dip your applicator to a depth of two inches into the wax, then wipe the wax off one side of the applicator. Starting on the front of the shin, halfway between the knee and the ankle, hold the applicator on the edge and swipe down the leg in a smooth fast stroke. This will distribute a thin, rather than thick, coating of wax. Repeat this step with a dip, wipe, and stroke until the lower half of the front of one leg is covered. Set your applicator down on the edge of the wax container. Now you are ready for the removal of wax and hair. Take a deep breath.

Removing the wax will not be terribly uncomfortable if you do it with quick removal strokes. It's the same principle as removing a Band-Aid: The slower you pull, the more painful it is. To remove the wax, you will need to apply your removal strip, or what I call a pick-up strip. If you are new to waxing, it will be more comfortable to use small strips. Smaller strips will remove less hair with each pull. The only drawback to this is that it will take longer. I always use small strips on a first-time "waxee" in my salon, even though it may cause me to run a little behind in my schedule. The slower I go with a beginner, the more likely that person will return for the service and continue to wax. After you get used to waxing, you can graduate to larger-size strips. A good-size strip to begin with is the exact size of a dollar bill. Cut your strips to that size.

To remove the wax, always start at the bottom of the leg and work your way up. You'll realize, after you've done a few removal strips, that this keeps your hands from getting sticky. To remove, place the strip on top of the wax and *gently* rub the strip two or three times in a downward stroke. Don't make the mistake that most professionals make in pressing the strip down hard. This is taught in schools for some reason and is absolutely wrong. By pressing hard, you will force the wax to stick more stringently to the skin, causing more pain and pulling on the skin. After the two or three soft strokes, lift up a small tab at the bottom of the strip closest to the ankle and pull quickly but smoothly up the leg. Voila! You should have a strip of smooth, hair-free skin. I hope you didn't find this too uncomfortable. The first time I had my legs waxed, I was a little shocked at how it felt. I will tell you that the first time was the only time that it smarted. After that, it was a piece of cake and I have never gone back to shaving.

Continue with the same strip to remove the rest of the wax on the front part of the lower half of your leg. You can continue using one strip to accomplish this until the strip gets really thick with wax. Discard and get another strip.

For the top half of the lower leg, continue with your leg out in front of you, applying the wax by starting just under the knee to the area that you just waxed. Apply three or four rows of wax first, put down your applicator, and then remove all the wax with a strip. To wax the knee area, bend your knee and place your foot flat on the ground. To wax properly, always pull skin tightly. Bending the knee helps to tighten the knee area. Apply the wax in small patches to accommodate the curve of the knee. Dip your applicator only one inch into the pot of wax. Remember to use the scraping technique; otherwise, the wax will be applied too thickly. A thinner application will remove the hair best. When removing the wax in the knee area, work with small strips because of the curved area. The knee area has coarser, tougher skin, making hair removal here relatively painless.

WAX YOURSELF NEW

Waxing is not only a beneficial hair-removal method, it also aids in exfoliation. After waxing your legs, your skin will be smooth and free of dead skin build-up.

The rest of your leg waxing will follow the same procedure as before. The only obstacle is tackling the difficulty of waxing the back of the calf area. You will figure out your own method, depending on your flexibility. Just remember to apply wax downward from the back of the knees to the Achilles tendon. Remove the wax by pulling up in the opposite direction. Waxing yourself is possible, but it may be more awkward for you than you wish to deal with. The inability to reach the tough spots is why most women seek the help of professionals. I personally do both, depending on what is most convenient. You may try waxing and may enjoy it, or you may just say "forget it" and make an appointment at a salon. Whatever the case, don't give up on waxing and go back to shaving. If you hang in there, I believe you'll be very happy later in life when you have a lot less body hair.

Waxing Other Body Areas

Based on my salon experience, here are the other areas of the body that are the most commonly waxed:

Lower legs

Upper legs

Bikini line

Forearms

Upper arms

Underarms

Hands and knuckles

Eyebrows

Upper lip

Chin

Sideburns and sides of the face

Lower Legs

The lower legs are relatively easy to wax yourself at home and I've just outlined the procedure for them. Waxing on the lower legs should be done every six to eight weeks.

Upper Legs

The upper legs are a toss-up when it comes to doing it yourself or in a salon because it is difficult to reach and see the hair on the backs of the upper thighs. I find that I can accomplish the backs of the thighs if I prop my foot up on the bathroom counter. You will be working sort of blindly back there, but it is not impossible. The fortunate thing is that hair is relatively sparse on the back of the thighs. Remember to protect your countertop with an old towel if you attempt this at home. You will probably need to wax your upper legs every six to eight weeks.

Bikini Line

Waxing the bikini area has grown in leaps and bounds in popularity over the last five years. Women have discovered that waxing this area relieves the discomfort of the rash associated with shaving the tender area that lies beneath our underwear. Good bikini waxes can alleviate hair for six weeks or more. This is a great reprieve from shaving. Many women are afraid to get a bikini wax because they imagine that it will be very painful. The remarkable thing is that this area along our panty line is fairly insensitive. If you think about it, you usually don't feel the presence of the elastic panty line. The other reason that a bikini wax is relatively painless is because the coarser hair that grows there is more easily removed than leg hair. You may be very surprised at how easy a bikini wax is to tolerate. You will also love the results.

I don't recommend giving yourself a bikini wax unless you are very good at waxing. This area is difficult to manage because you can't see way down under to remove all the hair. It is also difficult to hold the skin on the inside of the thigh tightly enough to remove the hair efficiently. The skin in the groin area can be thin and sensitive to the rapid pulling in the removal stage. It is very easy to bruise the skin when pulling. Have a professional bikini wax several times before you attempt this area. When you feel more comfortable, give it a try, using very small applications of wax. Remove this wax with small strips of pick-up material to ensure that you don't bruise the skin.

The newest waxing rage in salons today is the Brazilian bikini wax, named after the tiny thong bathing suit bottoms popular on Brazilian beaches. A Brazilian wax usually means that a lot of bikini hair is removed, just leaving a small strip of hair down the middle of the body. Some salons offer to remove all the hair entirely. This should always be done with a pair of thong panties on to protect the skin from dripping wax and for client modesty. The thong is usually shifted to accommodate hair removal. A true professional who is trained in this service will perform this request in a manner that is comfortable to the client. This service is not one I recommend unless you have been getting regular bikini waxes for a while. Removing that much hair is too difficult and tedious for a novice. Bikini waxes should be done every six to eight weeks.

Forearms

Removing hair from the forearms is very easy to do at home. You should follow the same procedure I described earlier. The only secret to the forearms is to pay attention to the direction in which the hair grows. You must apply the wax in the direction of the hair growth. Notice that the hair on your forearm wraps around the arm instead of growing down the arm. You should apply the wax in an arc around the arm and pull off the wax in an arc as well. The hair on your forearm is very fine and is usually painless to remove. Make sure to powder the arm very good with cornstarch to lessen the chance of pulling up on the skin. You will probably need to wax this area every eight to twelve weeks.

Upper Arms

Most of us don't grow a lot of hair on our upper arms, but some women have a fine, dark, furry layer on their upper arms, all the way up to the shoulders. Using a mirror, you could probably wax this area yourself. If you use a mirror to help see where to apply the wax, make sure you spread out towels to protect the countertop. Chances are, the mirror that you may use will be the one over your bathroom sink. For upper arms, remember to follow the hair growth in the wax application and remove against the growth. You will probably need to wax this area every eight to twelve weeks.

Underarms

Waxing the hair under your arms is not easy because you need both of your hands to hold the skin tightly while you pull the wax and hair off. I strongly recommend that you have this service done in a salon. The beauty of waxing the underarms is that the hair will diminish here rather quickly over the next several waxes. The hair becomes very soft when it returns and feels far better than the stubble that grows out after shaving. You may feel a little self-conscious about letting your hair grow out to have a wax service in the underarm area. Many women are embarrassed to have any amount of hair growing under their arms. Try to start waxing your underarms in the winter months, when sleeveless tops are rarely worn. By the summertime, you will have a lot less hair growing there. You will need to have an underarm wax every six to eight weeks.

Hands and Knuckles

Some of you may think I'm crazy to even mention this area, but you'd be surprised at how many women have dark, fine hair that grows on the back of the hands and knuckles. These areas are very easy and painless to wax. Use small dabs of wax on the knuckles and small strips to remove. Make a fist with the hand that is to be waxed to keep the skin tight when removing the wax. Make sure to apply the wax in the direction that the hair grows, probably down toward the fingertips. Remove the wax in the opposite direction. Make a fist while waxing the back of the hand as well. You will find that the fine hair on the hands and knuckles will return very slowly. You will probably need to wax these areas every eight to twelve weeks.

Eyebrows

Brow waxing is the most requested waxing service in salons; however, I don't recommend that waxing be done on the brows except for exceptionally bushy brows. The reason for this is because eyebrows require a lot of accuracy in removing the hair to create a perfect shape. I have dedicated an entire chapter to the eyebrows to help you with the details of this very important facial feature. Please read chapter 9 for my home secrets to perfect brow shaping.

If you do insist on waxing your brows, consult a good salon that is experienced in the proper brow-waxing technique. Not every licensed professional has an eye for great brow shaping. Seek out a recommendation from someone you know. When you go into a salon for your brow service, look at the brows of the person who will do the work (if it's a female). The way she wears her eyebrows will be a good indication of how she will wax yours. Beware of anyone with strange, over-tweezed, or trendy brows.

Close your eyes during this service to protect them from the cornstarch and wax. Waxing should be done with a tiny applicator such as a wooden orangewood stick. This will ensure the accuracy that is necessary for a perfect shape. The waxing should only be done to remove the very outer hairs of the brow line or the hairs that grow between the brows. The shaping of the brow should be developed with tweezers. The skin around the brows is very sensitive, so be sure that the person providing the waxing service applies a good dusting of cornstarch. Let's hope that the service provider doesn't press the removal strip over the wax with a lot of pressure. Don't be afraid to ask her to use very light pressure on your brow area. Never get a brow wax if you are using Retin-A on your skin. The use of Retin-A will likely cause the top layer of your skin to come off with the wax, resulting in a raw spot and later a scab.

I believe that a salon professional should teach home maintenance as part of the brow service. It's impossible to keep the brow area precise and clean-looking without tweezing a few hairs every few days. That's why it's important to know how to properly tweeze and shape your own brows. Ask the salon professional to teach you the guidelines. Many of them will be reluctant, because they want you to return only to them for this service. By now you should have read chapter 9, "In Search of the Perfect Brows." If so, you will be fine on your own.

Upper Lip

This is a very necessary part of every woman's personal grooming. Most women over age 25 have fine hair that grows above the lip. For many, this hair is pale and not that noticeable. For others, it is very dark and coarse, nearly like a man's mustache. I have had teens starting at age 12 come into the salon for their first lip wax. Many young women with darker hair are plagued with a mustache at a tender young age. The removal of this dark hair immediately raises the self-esteem of a young girl. If you start waxing the hair on the upper lip at a very young age, it will diminish on a permanent basis and virtually be nonexistent by the time you reach your 30s. I share the embarrassment many women feel from jokes commonly made about women with a mustache.

Waxing the hair on your upper lip is relatively easy, but this is one area of the body that is sensitive to hair removal. The first time you wax this area, you will be a little shocked at how it smarts. The quicker you pull off the removal strip, the easier it will be. If you're nervous about how much it will hurt, try to have your first lip wax done at a salon. Having someone else do it is a lot easier the first time around.

When you wax the upper lip, the secret is simply to use a very thick coating of cornstarch. The wax should be applied in two strokes. Start at the middle of the upper lip, and stroke to the outer corner of the lip on one side. Your second application will start from the middle of the upper lip and sweep to the other corner of the lip. Apply a small strip of muslin or paper bag material to one-half of the upper lip. Press lightly and stroke only one or two times from the middle to the outer corner. Lift the outer corner of the strip with one hand while holding the side of the lip tightly, pulling slightly toward the jaw. Remove the strip quickly and smoothly. The stinging sensation will pass quickly. Repeat the removal step for the other side. Your upper lip may tingle for as long as 20 minutes. It is common for the upper lip to get red for a few hours, so don't get too nervous. After a few hours and the redness subsides, I recommend applying a topical antiseptic like Sea Breeze. This will help prevent breakouts from lip waxing. If you experience a breakout after lip waxing, note that this will usually occur only the first few times the hair is removed. Most women I've waxed rarely have this breakout experience, but because I've seen it happen several times, I feel it is worth mentioning. You will need to wax this area every six to eight weeks.

Chin

Oh, why do we females have to grow hair on our chinny-chin-chin? I have no idea, except that most often it is due to the slow-down of female hormones after age 30. The estrogen starts to taper off, allowing the male hormones in our body to influence the sudden sprouting of hair in the chin area. Only about 30 percent of women need to wax their chins. If you haven't noticed any dark or heavy hair in that area, you should feel lucky. The nice thing about the chin area is that it is not very sensitive, so hair removal here is painless. The hair usually grows in a downward direction on the chin. You can give yourself a chin wax relatively easily. Simply dust the chin area with a coating of cornstarch. Apply the wax with a Popsicle stick from the front of the chin, down and under. You will probably need to apply three small dabs. Using a small strip, press lightly over the wax downward and remove in an upward pulling motion. Removal should be done in three small sections. Your chin will probably not tingle or get red. You will need to wax the chin area every eight to twelve weeks.

Sideburns and Sides of the Face

Some women have sideburn hair that makes them feel uncomfortable. Dark, fine hair can grow from the sideburn area down and all over the cheeks. I recommend that you go to a salon to have this properly treated, for the simple reason that it is difficult to see what you are doing in this area. Many women want their entire faces waxed because they are uncomfortable with the fine peach fuzz they have on their faces. The only problem with removing all the hair on the face is that this will make the skin look fairly unnatural. A face without soft, downy hair tends to look plastic and shiny, almost like a mannequin. Be careful to remove just the hair that is dark and coarse. A beautiful complexion will always have the presence of fine hair. Don't get obsessive about having a completely bald face. You will regret having your face completely waxed. Waxing the entire face also leads to breakouts. It is not a good trade-off.

Waxing for Men

I WANTED TO INCLUDE this section for men because men always call the salon and ask about waxing services. Most men call to inquire about waxing their faces so that they won't have to shave. The hair on a man's face is far too coarse to remove with wax. The density would also make it extremely painful, so I don't recommend it. The second-most requested waxing service for men is back waxing. For men who have an excessive amount of hair on their backs, waxing is a wonderful treatment to have done. Even the hairiest of men can enjoy sporting a clean-looking, hairless back after frequent waxing treatments. One of my male customers had an extremely hairy back and was embarrassed to go swimming in the summertime. After two years of waxing his back every other month, his hair was diminished by 60 percent. Now he waxes only every three or four months. Eventually, he will not have to wax at all. Many men would like to have the hair on their backs gone, but are modest about coming into a salon to have it waxed. Waxing at home may be the ideal solution for a man who is embarrassed about the hair on his back. You may have a spouse, boyfriend, or family member who might appreciate a back wax at home.

The back is fairly sensitive, so make sure that a lot of cornstarch is used before applying the wax. Work in small sections so that the waxing will be comfortable. The skin may become very red after the treatment, but this should subside after a few hours. Applying an antiseptic to the skin will aid in the prevention of breakouts. A back wax should probably be done every eight to twelve weeks.

The body-building craze has created the need for chest and complete body waxing for men. The waxing process for men is just like the one for women. Just follow these three simple rules:

1. Use lots of cornstarch to create a barrier between the skin and the wax
2. Apply wax in the direction of the hair growth
3. Remove the hair against the hair growth

Other Things to Know About Waxing

HERE ARE THE FINER points about waxing that will make you a pro. Whether you do it yourself at home or have the service done in a salon, you'll benefit from knowing the rest of my waxing secrets.

Ingrown Hairs

The only drawback to waxing, in my opinion, is that waxing can cause the occurrence of ingrown hairs. This is because the hair that regenerates from the roots is sometimes blocked by dead skin cells as the hair begins to bud at the surface of the skin. This appearance of the hair at the surface usually occurs one to two weeks after the waxing service. You'll usually feel slightly itchy, or a tingling sensation, when the hair begins to emerge from beneath the skin. This is your signal to exfoliate vigorously on a daily basis in the bath or shower. You can use a loofah sponge or an exfoliating mitt, along with a body scrub. I recommend one of my body scrubs, described in chapter 13, "Spa at Home" (my favorite is sugar and oil). The idea is to keep the skin's surface free of the dry skin cell build-up to help the hairs resurface freely. If you do a good job at exfoliation, you will have no problem with ingrown hairs.

Post-Waxing Rash

Immediately after waxing, your skin may be covered with tiny red bumps, as if you have the measles. Don't be alarmed. These "measles" are actually a good sign, although annoying if you waxed right before a trip to the pool. The red spots mark each hair that was properly removed from the root. The redness may be accompanied by a slight goosebump. Your skin may look like the skin of a plucked chicken. Essentially, that's what just happened to your skin. Your "feathers" were plucked. The redness and bumps may last for 24 to 48 hours, so be prepared. The trauma to the root will deter the hair from growing back, and eventually the hairs will die.

After Waxing

To clean up the residue that might be left on the skin, simply wipe the area with a damp towel if you used my homemade sugar wax. If you used a commercial tree resin wax, do not use the cleanser that may have come with the wax kit. I have found these cleansers to be irritating to some skin types. All you need to use to clean up resin wax is vegetable oil. Massage the oil into the skin and wipe it off with a damp towel. Wait a couple of hours to apply any lotions or moisturizers. This will allow the follicle or the pore to close back down and prevent irritation.

If you take a bath or shower immediately after a leg, bikini, or arm wax, use warm water at first, then boost the temperature up to the hot level that you like. The open follicles will make the skin slightly more sensitive to extremely warm temperatures.

SOOTHING THE SKIN

Waxing has never bothered my skin in the least, but some individuals get quite red and report a rashy, itchy feeling after waxing. This may be due to the resin wax that is used, or perhaps their skin is just sensitive because the hair was removed. I recommend a topical, 2-percent hydrocortisone cream, which may be purchased at any drugstore. Apply the cream immediately following the waxing and for a couple of days until the skin feels normal.

Baby Steps

I BELIEVE THAT WAXING is the most excellent way to remove hair, but it's not for everyone. Try it in baby steps, starting with an upper lip wax or lower leg wax in a good salon. As you see the results and get more comfortable, you may just end

WAXING CAUTION!

Never have a waxing service done at a salon or by yourself just before a big event unless you are experienced with the way your skin will react. For instance, don't have your upper lip waxed the day before your wedding if you've never done it before or are not sure how your skin will respond. I have had women come in for a bikini wax the day before they left on a cruise. I always discourage them if it's their first time because they might find that they will be too red for the next few days.

· 12 ·
Beauty in a Blink

*"You will never find time for anything.
If you want time, you must make it."* CHARLES BIXTON

THE BEAUTY TIPS in this chapter will help you get out your front door each day looking fabulous, even when you're short on time. Being busy doesn't mean you can't look beautiful. I'll teach you how to get ahead of the clock so your appearance doesn't have to take a back seat to your schedule.

When I first started working in a salon, I became acutely aware of time in relationship to beauty. In the beginning, all I focused on was how to make someone more beautiful. Which tools should I use? How should I cut the hair? Where should I put the blush? What shade of red would look best in this person's hair? But my concerns were secondary to the clients' main concern: "How much time will it take to get that look?"

More often than not, when I consulted with clients, the first words they spoke were, "I want a new look, but I don't have a lot of time to get ready." Or, "I need something that's low maintenance." A stylist can give anyone a low-maintenance cut. After all, shaving the head is a low-maintenance hairstyle, but not many women would go for it. The point is, why not have the style you really want and be smart about fitting it into your life? If you determine that looking good is important, then you need to organize yourself enough to pull it off. Let's assume you want to look your best every day, not just for special occasions. Making it happen means making it a habit. It's no different than getting a cup of coffee every morning or brushing your teeth. Once you've decided that your beauty routine is important enough, making it a habit will become natural to you. Step One is deciding to *do it!*

You've already learned Step Two: how to make yourself beautiful. By now, you know the ABCs of hairstyling, makeup, skin care, and so on. Step Three is to organize all the ABCs into a natural order that will save you time. You may be amazed how little time it takes to look great.

First, analyze what you do with your time at present. Make a timeline of your current activities in the morning. If you work, what time do you wake up and what time do you leave the house for your job? If you have just 30 minutes, from taking a shower to grabbing your car keys, then you'll have to learn to work more efficiently than most, but it can be done. I'm not the busiest person in the world, but I have a lot on my plate. I have a business that's open seven days a week, I juggle two TV shows, and I raise two children alone. Time is precious and can feel like the enemy much of the time. Sometimes on crazy chaotic mornings, I may want to sacrifice the time it takes to beautify myself. My job requires that I look the part, so I've had to find a way to do it all. Here are my personal solutions to a crunched time schedule.

Being highly organized is the key. At first, my suggestions may seem difficult to accomplish. Give them a try, one step at a time. Your rewards will be apparent right off the bat. The first reward will be your reflection in the mirror. Others will take notice, including co-workers, family, and friends. Positive comments from others will feed your own self-motivation. The steps toward your new routine will quickly become a habit instead of a chore.

Motivations

BEFORE YOU DIVE INTO a new routine, you may find it helpful to feed your motivation. Think of some reasons for putting forth a good image or impression. Remember what it was like to prepare for your first job interview? Would you dream of applying for your first job without looking your best? Of course not, but after we land a job, isn't it easy to slip into a routine of going to work half put-together? The first day on the job, everyone puts forth a good effort. Imagine getting up each day as if it is your first day at work. Here are some other motivations:

1. Pretend each day that you are getting ready for your first date with someone you're really anxious to go out with.
2. Pretend you are giving a speech that day in front of a big audience.
3. Pretend you are giving a big presentation to your boss and co-workers.
4. Pretend that you have a lunch date with a friend you haven't seen in a long time.
5. Pretend that you're going to run into your "ex."
6. Pretend that you are meeting your husband or wife for a date after work.
7. Pretend that you are a news anchor. Your job depends on viewer ratings.
8. Pretend you are going to your high school reunion.

I love the last one because high school reunions are a huge motivation for women to come to a salon for a makeover. The thought of meeting up with old school mates highly motivates people to want to look their best. Imagining these scenarios creates what I call "beauty adrenaline." This adrenaline energizes us to take extra steps toward looking great.

All of these motivators can be channeled into a daily game of inspiration. Do whatever it takes to make the routine in the morning more joyful. You will have greater success in accomplishing the ultimate goal of making a good impression. It is no different than what a marathon runner does to prepare for a race. It's a mind game.

Get Organized

EVERY ONCE IN A while, a client dashes into my salon after work to fix up for an evening function. I work downtown in a busy metropolitan center, where there are restaurants and theaters. My clients know that they can come in to get ready, either with my help or on their own. When I invite them to use the makeup bar or my hair station, they always comment on how fast they can get ready there. The reason it's easier for them at the salon than at their home is because the tools and work area are very organized. Everything they need is at their fingertips. That's my first secret to helping you get ready in a blink. You need to organize your bathroom at home to function as smoothly as a professional salon. The biggest positive outcome from this is that getting ready will be more fun and you'll accomplish it more smoothly.

Most women have too much stuff. We are shoppers by nature and seem to collect a ton of things as a result. The truth is, it takes a lot of time every day to sort through all the "stuff" to find what we need. Take a look at men for a moment. When a man travels, his overnight bag consists of a razor, a blow dryer, a toothbrush, and a comb. Men get ready for the day in 20 minutes or less. Of course, they don't have to deal with a makeup bag, but makeup should add only 10 minutes to your "get ready" time. Men have to shave their faces each day, so that is about the equivalent of a woman's "makeup" time. Men just deal with things more efficiently when getting ready. I learned a lot by observing the way men get ready. They just open a drawer and get the job done.

The first step is organizing your bathroom to set up what you need in three groups:

1. Shelf for face and body cosmetics
2. Hair basket or drawer
3. Makeup bag or drawer

In the medicine cabinet, line up your facial moisturizer, body lotion, deodorant, and whatever else you use, like contact lens solution. Don't mix in any hair products. Keep items lined up in the order that you will apply them. Next, establish where you'll organize your hair necessities. This can be in a drawer, if you have one, or a wicker basket. Put in the basket only what you use on a daily basis. Remove everything else that you've collected and store these items in a different place for occasional use. Your daily basket should include one styling brush, one comb, and two or three bottles of styling product, spray, and so forth. The idea is to "see and grab" exactly what you need to get the job done. This will make it easy to get things out and put things away.

When it comes to makeup, most women keep an abundant amount of makeup in a bag so that they can take everything with them. This wastes time. I use a different approach. At home I have a basket of makeup that I use to get ready with. I also have small bag of touch-up items I keep in my car. I never co-mingle them. This keeps everything less cluttered and makes it easier to see the items, which keeps the steps of putting on your makeup flowing smoothly.

A touch-up kit can be accessible in your car or at work. My single most important piece of advice here is to stop collecting! Keep what you have narrowed down to only what you need. You can do a great job of making yourself up in 10 minutes or less. If spending

DRINK IT UP

Include an extra five minutes in the morning to prepare a cup of tea or coffee for yourself. I find that getting ready in the morning is more pleasant if I take the time to prepare a beverage.

only 10 minutes seems impossible, refer to chapter 8, "De-Mystifying Makeup."

Shower or Bath Organization

Here's another area where we girls tend to clutter up the works. Try to limit the stuff in your shower to just the items you use every day. The basics should include one bottle of shampoo, one bottle of conditioner, your body cleanser, an exfoliating mitten, and perhaps a razor if you shave your legs. I keep a toothbrush in the shower even though I have one at the sink. I love to brush my teeth in the shower while my hair conditioner is soaking in.

Clothing

My best secret to getting dressed in a hurry is to have my outfit ready the night before. I used to get my boys' clothing out for the next day at their bedtime and lay out everything for them like a little body on the floor. Shirt, pants, undies, socks, and shoes helped me create the little figure on the carpet at the foot of their beds. In the morning when they got up, they could dress themselves even at a young age, and there was no chaos about deciding what to wear. For adults, the concept is the same, but instead of the floor layout, I recommend that you hang up the outfit on the back of your bedroom or bathroom door. Try to get everything ready that you will need, even panty hose or socks and shoes. Hang the belt or scarf on the hanger. I even loop the bra and panties I will wear on the hanger, and they're the first things I grab in the morning after my shower. I find that I'm much more able to put the look together at night than in the morning when I'm a little groggy. You can even get in the habit of assembling the ensemble at the same time you undress from work. The morning will be a breeze if you get your act together the night before.

Ready, Set, Go!

Okay, here's the routine. I've received many congratulations from family and friends who are amazed at how quickly I can get out the door in the morning. I think most of my skills were learned from my days of working as a ramp model. Changing backstage between appearances sometimes took just two minutes. I got used to being a quick-change artist.

My order of events is as follows:

1. Shower, wash, and condition hair; brush teeth (5 to 8 minutes)
2. Step out, dry off, and apply face and body moisturizer (2 minutes)
3. Dry and style hair while your body is wrapped in a towel or robe (10 minutes, maybe 15, if your hair is very long)
4. Apply your makeup (8 to 10 minutes)
5. Get dressed (5 minutes)

The things that add time to your schedule are shaving your legs and drying long hair. I don't shave; I wax my legs once a month. If you decide to start waxing at a salon, or take advantage of chapter 11, "The Secrets of Waxing," you will love the freedom of not having to shave your legs or underarms every day. If you do choose to shave your legs, you can save time by doing it while your hair conditioner is on.

You may also consider shaving at night in a warm bath. It won't seem like such a chore if you enjoy a spa bath ritual at the same time. If you have long hair, also consider washing your hair at night during the shaving time. Your hair can finishing drying completely overnight and just need a little run-through in the morning with a blow dryer and brush.

SPEED IT UP

For a speedy start for your makeup application, try to select a creme foundation with a sponge applicator. The coverage is better, and applying a foundation of this type is swift and easy.

Your hairstyling and makeup routine has been clearly outlined for you in earlier chapters of this book. At first you may not be as speedy as I've recommended, but you'll get faster in no time. Always put each item you use back in its proper place, and never set the bottles or tools on the counter. I learned this from a dermatologist I used to know. He was German and very efficient. The idea is to never put something away twice. Take a cream down from the shelf, get out what you need from the jar, and then put the jar back on the shelf. You'll never waste any time on clean-up.

Some of you may find that it makes more sense to put on your makeup before you style your hair. That's perfectly fine; just reverse the order of those two steps. I use my hair-drying time to let my facial moisturizer dry before putting on makeup. You'll figure out what is best for you.

After dressing, off you go. Remember that you have a small touch-up kit of makeup in your car. When you arrive at work, freshen up your lipstick, but *not while driving, please!* I always get a cup of coffee on the way to work, so the lipstick touch-up is a definite must for me.

More Tips for Beauty in a Blink

1. Don't wash your hair every single day. Every other day cleansing is suitable for most people. On the day that you don't wash your hair, simply restyle quickly with brush and blow dryer, or set your hair in self-adhering rollers *before* you get in the shower. The steam from the shower will give you a great style.

2. Stick to the same order every day when applying your makeup. Don't bounce around the face and get lost in what you're doing. After applying foundation, start at the eyebrows and work your way down.

3. Keep your clothing simple. Don't get hung up on presenting an endless variety of outfits. Most people won't remember what you wear from one day to the next.

4. Have a clock in your bathroom. Play a little game with yourself about how long it takes to get ready. Push yourself a little and don't let your mind wander.

Be Consistent

This chapter gave you some tips on how to be efficient when getting ready. If you can convince yourself that looking beautiful can happen in a short amount of time, you will stay on the beauty track. Knowing what to do is half the battle. Doing it every day will be your victory!

· 13 ·

Spa at Home

"When we get too caught up in the busyness of the world, we lose connection with one another— and ourselves." JACK KORNFIELD

$\mathcal{M}$Y LOVE AFFAIR with day spas began in 1985 while living in Europe during my modeling career. The Europeans were already enjoying a lifestyle full of self-indulgence and relaxation, including massage, pedicures, and facials. The birth of the urban spa soon caught on in the United States. Americans began to branch out from the obligatory monthly haircut to more pleasurable experiences, and day spas started cropping up all over the country.

I opened my first day spa in 1988, offering everything from massage to waxing. I soon realized that people were hungry for relaxation, due to their hectic schedules, and couldn't always make time to come in for spa treatments. I created the concept of "spa at home" for many of our regular clients by teaching massage for couples and aromatherapy classes.

In this book, I teach many of the spa techniques I've developed over the years in my day spas. You'll have a rewarding experience doing these treatments for yourself and sharing them with family and friends. Before we actually begin, let's delve into massage and aromatherapy, the cornerstones of the spa industry.

Massage

THERE IS A FAMOUS saying in the massage business, "Even a bad massage is still heavenly." I don't agree completely with that statement, but the inference is that all massage feels good. Massage has been around since ancient times and may be defined as a systematic form of touch that comforts, soothes, and promotes good health. Massage is the oldest and simplest of all medical treatments. It provides not only physical benefits, but psychological ones as well.

BENEFITS OF MASSAGE

There are so many benefits of massage. Massage increases circulation and venous flow to the heart, lowers blood pressure, relaxes tight muscles and muscle spasms, increases the percentage of oxygen in the tissues, helps eliminate waste from the body, helps stimulate lymphatic flow, and aids in the removal of lactic acid in the muscles following a strenuous workout.

Psychological benefits rate even higher in my book. Most of us need to be touched. Medical research has shown that infants who are not cuddled or stroked often fail to thrive at the normal rate. The same is true for adults. Our mental well being is elevated when massage is received. Massage is beneficial psychologically to both the receiver and the giver. When receiving massage, one may feel comforted, soothed, relaxed, euphoric, nurtured, and calm. Givers of massage will also feel a deep sense of relaxation and calmness, knowing that they are administering the pleasure of massage.

You've Been Massaging All Along

If you think about it, you're already an accomplished massage thera-pist. From the time we're children, we learn to perform massage on ourselves. When you had a fall as a child, what did your parent tell you to do? Rub it, right? How about that Charlie-horse you got in your calf on the school playground? I'll bet you learned quickly how to knead it until it relaxed. Have you ever rubbed a headache away by applying circular strokes to your temples? The list goes on. So, you've got a head start at self-massage. Now, you just need a little education in some new techniques that you can use on others.

Getting Started

As you delve into learning the art of massage, imagine you are the giver and the receiver, throughout each step. As you learn technique, imag-ine how the movements would feel. This will develop your intuition to deliver the proper touch, pressure, and strokes.

Consult Your Physician

Before receiving a massage, be sure to consult a doctor about any phys-ical problems you may have that might be aggravated by massage. People with back or neck injuries, joint problems, or circulatory ail-ments should be very cautious about receiving a massage, especially from beginners.

The Giver

To properly give someone a massage, wear comfortable clothing, wash your hands, and make sure that your fingernails are short and smooth. You should remove any wrist or finger jewelry.

The Receiver

To receive a massage, dress in loose clothing such as shorts and an un-dershirt, or, if you feel comfortable, you can receive a massage without clothing. You may choose to have a sheet or blanket over your body that can be shifted out of the way for each part of the body as it's being massaged. It is important to be warm, so I recommend receiving a massage with a blanket covering your body.

Equipment

Many families and couples who are into massage invest in a traditional massage table. Tables can run from $150 to $600. Don't despair if you can't afford this, as massage can be performed on the floor, on a firm mattress, or even in a recliner. You should consider using old sheets and blankets during a massage because these may be stained with oils or lotions.

Oils and Lotions

I prefer oil over lotion when giving a massage, for the simple reason that oils tend to lubricate the skin and keep the body warm. The moisture in lotions evaporates and can make you feel cold. (This is beneficial if you have the tendency to get hot, as the lotion will keep you cooler.) Any body lotion will do.

Oils may be mixed in different combinations for a different slip. I recommend good old canola oil because it's fairly lightweight, washes out of sheets and clothing, and is easy to shower off. If you want to do a little shopping, try mixing equal parts canola oil, grapeseed oil, and sweet almond oil. (This is the blend we use in my day spa.)

Your oil or lotion should be stored in a dark bottle to filter out light. It is easier to dispense during massage in a flip-top bottle, rather than a pump. I recommend an 8-ounce bottle, since it's easier to grip when your hands are lubricated.

Some ABCs

Massage is simply the compression of a muscle between your hand and the bones or tissues that lie under that muscle. The compression is done by moving parts of your hands over the muscle. You will use four parts of your hand when giving a basic massage: the heel, thumbs, fingers, and the entire hand. The most important aspects to consider when giving a massage are which part of the hand to use for a certain stroke, how much pressure to use, and the speed in which the stroke is performed relative to that pressure. For instance, if you do a stroke and use light pressure, the speed of the stroke may be faster than the speed of a stroke using hard pressure. *Use slow speed for deep pressure; use faster speed for light pressure.* How will you know how much pressure is the right amount? Ask. When you first begin to give a massage, ask your partner how the pressure is. Communication is the key. As you give more massages, you'll graduate to a level of intuition in which you can judge the pressure by how your partner responds. If the person jerks, winces, or fidgets during a stroke, the pressure is probably too great. If the person's muscles remain tight or the breathing pattern doesn't slow down, your pressure is probably too light and needs to be increased.

Direction of Strokes

In massage school a great deal of time is spent teaching students about the muscles and their attachments, hence which direction to work over the muscles. Most instructors teach you to massage toward the heart to deliver venous blood back to the heart and to receive new oxygen from the lungs. I've always felt strongly about massaging muscles in both directions, for there is a benefit to delivering freshly oxygenated blood to the tissues. In a nutshell, massage compresses muscles and stimulates the circulatory system. For that reason, you will learn strokes that move in both directions over muscles, arms, legs, and torso.

Solo Practice

Before massaging someone else, it's a good idea to practice some pressure techniques. Once you've mastered this, you'll be better equipped to start administering massage to others.

Basic Strokes and Pressure

For this exercise you just need your own dry hands. To understand how much pressure to use on the receiver, begin with developing a squeeze technique. With your right hand, squeeze your left thumb. Pretend that your thumb is frozen and your job is to knead it back to a soft, warm state simply by squeezing it. Next, move on to all of the fin-

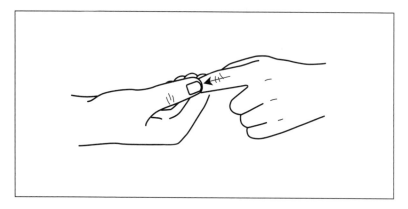

Figure 17. Firmly squeeze the finger between the index finger and your thumb, sliding and squeezing until you get to the tip of the finger.

gers on your left hand individually. You may be surprised to find that your fingers can take quite a bit of pressure.

Now, start at the base of each finger where the finger meets the hand and firmly squeeze the finger between the index finger and your thumb, sliding and squeezing until you get to the tip of the finger (see figure 17). As you pass over the joints or knuckles, you'll notice that it feels better to lighten up the pressure briefly.

Next, turn the palm of your left hand toward the ceiling. Pretend that the palm of your left hand is the face of a clock. The base of the thumb will be the eight o'clock position. Now apply squeezes with your right thumb on the palm and all of your right fingers under the back of your hand. Squeeze as you rotate clockwise around the entire palm of your left hand (see figure 18). This exercise is designed to help you understand how much pressure is comfortable to receive on the palm of your hand.

Repeat this entire hand exercise with a little lotion or oil. You'll notice that it takes a little coordination once you've added the lubrication.

Try it on your partner's hands, first without lotion or oil, then with lotion or oil. Make sure your partner tells you if you need to increase or decrease the pressure.

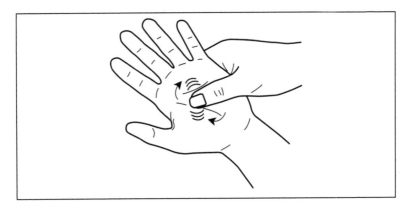

Figure 18. With the base of your thumb at the eight o'clock position of your palm, apply squeezes with your right thumb on the palm and all of your right fingers under the back of your hand. Squeeze as you rotate clockwise around the entire palm of your left hand.

Types of Strokes

Before you actually start to massage your partner, let's establish a language of strokes.

Squeezing Stroke

Use this on fingers, toes, forearms, wrists, and ankles. The entire hand or just the fingers wrap around the body part and squeeze. You can slide and squeeze to travel along the body part.

Kneading Stroke

This is mostly done by the thumbs working in a circular motion against the fingers. Kneading moves are generally done going toward the heart on the feet, hands, arms, and legs.

Gliding Stroke

It is easy to get the hang of gliding strokes. You will generally use the entire hand from palm to fingertips, in a flat to slightly cupped position. Gliding strokes should be performed with deeper pressure and slower speed. You will use gliding strokes especially for larger muscles and areas of the body, such as the back, buttocks, chest, thighs, and arms.

HAND AND ARM MASSAGE

I always teach couples massage by starting with an arm and hand massage. I encourage you to tackle this first because this massage is performed face-to-face, and givers will be able to receive communication from their partners about pressure. It is important for givers to get feedback about their massage technique in order to gain confidence. Once you are confident about your strokes, you can begin to apply other techniques to other parts of the body.

To begin, have the receiver sit in an armchair or a recliner. The giver should sit to the side of the recipient, facing the opposite direction. Place a towel over the arm of the chair for protection. Apply a good amount of lubricant to the receiver's forearm and hand with a smooth, medium pressure, using a gliding stroke. Use both hands, with open palm, and compress the arm in-between your hands as you slide up and down the arm, applying the lubricant.

Where you start the massage is entirely up to you. I prefer to start with the hand. Using your thumbs, work the top of the hand with slow circular kneading strokes, using medium pressure. Be sure to lighten up a little bit when passing over the bones and knuckles.

Next, work on the fingers and thumb. Squeeze and slide one finger at a time, starting at the base of the finger and working your way down to the tip. Pause briefly at the tip of each finger for a slow squeeze. Now add a pulling stroke. With each finger, start at the base and squeeze and pull with good pressure, very slowly out to the tip. Finish by sliding off the tip of each finger. This will feel like you are emptying an upside-down tube of toothpaste by squeezing out every last bit.

Now, rotate the palm of the hand up to the ceiling. Use your thumbs on the palm and stroke in a circular kneading motion all over the palm. Pull and squeeze the fingers and thumb again. It feels fabulous with the hand rotated up; the giver's thumb can compress the meaty part of the fingers and thumb this way.

Now you're ready to proceed up the forearm. Hold the wrist in one hand and use the other hand to glide up the forearm and down again. Each time you glide up the arm, apply pressure between your thumb and the rest of your fingers. When I'm doing this large arm "glide," I think about pushing a very tight sleeve up the arm, and on the return stroke, I'm pulling the tight sleeve back down. When you've completed this glide three or four times, add some circular kneading strokes with your thumbs in the same up-and-down glide pattern, glide up the arm with thumbs circling, and down the arms with the fingers circling. Don't be discouraged if your hands are very tired at this point. Massage requires very strong hands, especially for the kneading strokes. Your hands will get stronger with time. If you get a cramp, shake it out gently, then continue, or better yet, have your partner give you a hand massage.

Above the Elbow

Use the same strokes you used on the forearm to work on the arm above the elbow. Anchor the arm of the receiver at the crook of the arm with one hand, while the other hand massages from the elbow to the top of the shoulder.

Counter Pressure in an Armchair

One reason I love to give an arm and hand massage in an armchair or recliner is because you can deliver some really great massage techniques by utilizing the arm of the chair. Lay the receiver's forearm on the arm of the chair, with the receiver's hand open and flat, palm facing down. Now, start at the receiver's wrist and glide up the forearm with the open palm of your hand, very slowly with deep pressure. Compress the forearm between your palm and the chair. Return back down to the wrist by squeezing the fingers around the forearm and pulling. Once you've mastered this, try going up the forearm again and continue to the shoulder, pushing the palm of your hand against the upper arm and squeezing back down. This big stroke feels great; repeat it as many as four or five times to finish the arm massage. This series of movements may be performed again on the arm with the palm turned up. Massaging the inside of the forearm will make the receiver's arm total spaghetti!

Don't forget to switch sides and massage the other hand and arm—I'm sure your partner will remind you.

FOOT AND LEG MASSAGE IN A CHAIR OR RECLINER

Now we're ready to move on to the feet and legs! The movements are very much the same as those used in the arm massage. The receiver should wear shorts or a bathrobe to expose the legs to the top of the thigh. You (the giver) should sit on a low stool at the foot of the chair or recliner or kneel on the floor on a pillow to protect your knees. Place a towel under the receiver's feet and legs to protect the recliner. If you use an armchair, you'll need to prop the feet and legs of the receiver on a stool or ottoman.

Remember that some people are very ticklish on their feet. If this is the case with the receiver, start first by just holding the foot firmly with your entire hand. Hold for five seconds, release, and hold again. Keep releasing and holding until your partner starts to relax. Being ticklish is usually a response to tense muscles. The squeezing technique will generally calm even the most ticklish feet. Each time you start a movement on the feet, use firm pressure and slow movements.

Start the foot massage by applying oil or lotion to your hands first, then very slowly applying it to the first foot. Begin with your thumbs on top of the foot, fingers wrapped under the arch of the foot. Work the thumbs in a circular motion and apply firm pressure, still keeping your fingers underneath (see figure 19). If your fingers move a lot with this movement, you may find your partner getting ticklish. Your thumbs should travel in circles from the base of the toes up to the ankle and back down (see figure 20). Squeeze and slide as you return to the toes. Try to change travel positions to the top and both sides of the foot as you pass up and down.

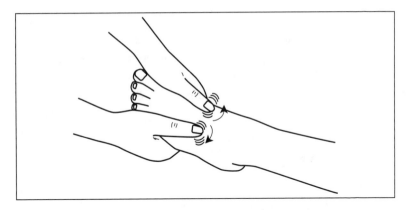

Figure 19. Starting with your thumbs on top of the foot and fingers wrapped under the arch of the foot, work the thumbs in a circular motion and apply firm pressure, still keeping your fingers underneath the foot.

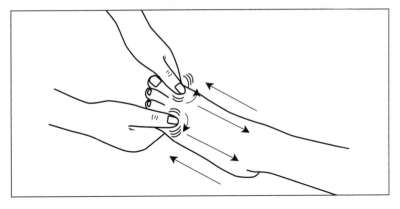

Figure 20. Move your thumbs in circles from the base of the toes up to the ankle and back down.

Now you are ready to concentrate on the toes individually. On each toe, use your thumb and index finger and make small circular movements, pulling down from the base of the toe to the tip (see figure 21). Squeeze and pull as you slide off the tip of each toe. Repeat for each toe, spending a little extra time on the big toe.

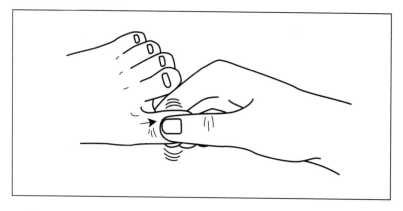

Figure 21. On each toe, use your thumb and index finger and make small circular movements, pulling down from the base of the toe to the tip.

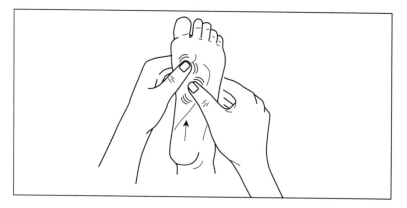

Figure 22. Make slow circular movements with your thumbs from the heel up the arch to the soles of the foot.

Bottoms of the Feet

This movement should be done very slowly, with a deliberate, even pressure so as not to tickle your partner. Change your hand position so that your thumbs are on the bottom side of the heel and your fingers are wrapped on top of the foot. Make slow circular movements with your thumbs from the heel up the arch to the soles of the foot (see figure 22).

As you travel up the foot, think about squeezing the foot between your fingers and thumbs. You should be using both of your hands on one of your partner's feet. While traveling up and down the foot, continue to circle with your thumbs in a smooth, constant motion.

Traveling Up the Legs

To accomplish the lower leg massage while the receiver is in the recliner, you will probably have to be up on your knees and leaning slightly forward. Starting at the ankle, use both of your hands and make large circular movements, with your thumbs on top of the leg and fingers underneath the leg, squeezing as you make your circles (see figure 23). Travel up the leg much as you did on the forearm. When you get to the knee, squeeze and slowly glide back down with a pulling motion. Each time you travel up the lower leg, change the path slightly to massage all parts of the leg and calf. Think about trying to push up the leg of very tight pants and then smoothing the pants back down again. Your thumbs should be on top of the shin and your fingers wrapped around under the calf as you pull back down to the ankle.

Massaging the thigh is difficult in a recliner unless you stand up, so we'll save instructions for that until we get to the floor massage.

MASSAGING THE BODY

The best place to massage the body at home is on the floor, using a couple of blankets to pad the floor surface. On top of the blankets, place an old sheet for protection from the oils and lotion. The receiver should lie down, face upward, to receive the chest, neck, and shoulder massage. Cover the receiver with a sheet and then a blanket if warmth is needed. Fold the sheet down to the chest, exposing the receiver's shoulders, head, and arms. You should sit or kneel above the receiver's head, facing the receiver's body (you'll be looking at them upside down). Apply oil or lotion to your hands and begin with gliding strokes to apply the lubricant across the chest, around the shoulders, and down the arms.

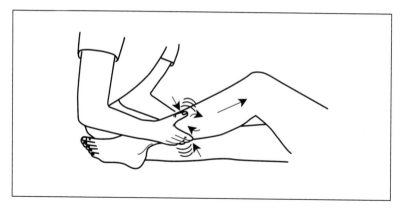

Figure 23. Starting at the ankle, use both of your hands and make large
circular movements, with your thumbs on top of the leg and fingers
underneath the leg, squeezing as you make your circles.

Chest

Extend your arms out straight in front of you, elbows straight, and
place the flat palm of your hands with fingers pointing toward the feet
of the receiver, directly on the chest just above the breasts. Your
thumbs should be tucked in against your hands; both thumbs will be
touching each other (see figure 24). Now lean down on the chest with
medium pressure and glide outward toward the shoulders. As you
reach the shoulders, wrap your fingers around the curve of the shoulders and keep gliding under the trapezius muscle, keeping your hands
open and flat. To complete this move, you will end up with your hands
meeting together behind the neck (see figure 25). Lift your hands up,
flip your hands over, and return to the beginning position on the chest
to repeat again. This is a very relaxing movement for the receiver and
should be performed several times. On the third or fourth pass keep
your hands under the neck for the next move.

Neck

Cup both of your hands under the neck, and slightly lift it up as if you
are raising the head, but don't cause the head to rise off the floor. Apply

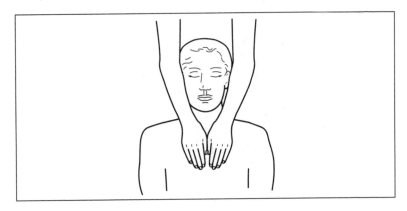

Figure 24. Extend your arms out straight in front of you, elbows straight, and place the flat palm of your hands with fingers pointing toward the feet of the receiver, directly on the chest just above the breasts. Your thumbs should be tucked in against your hands; both thumbs will be touching each other.

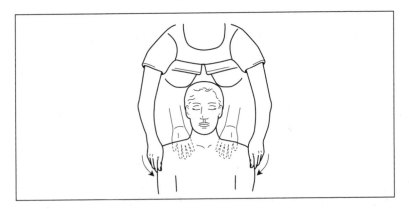

Figure 25. As you reach the shoulders, wrap your fingers around the curve of the shoulders and keep gliding under the trapezius muscle, keeping your hands open and flat. You will end up with your hands meeting together behind the neck.

pressure for a count of three, then relax. Now hold the receiver's head in your hands and gently and slowly roll the head to each side. This will release the muscles on each side of the neck.

Now imagine that you are typing on a keyboard, but you are doing so under the back of the neck with slow, firm pressure. You are exerting tapping-like pressure from the tips of your fingers to the back of the neck, from the top of the spine to the base of the head.

Shoulders

You (the giver) are still sitting or kneeling behind the receiver's head, facing the body. Place your hands on the round part of the shoulders, thumbs underneath, with your fingers pointing down the length of the arms (see figure 26). Simply press each shoulder, one at a time, toward the feet of the receiver (see figure 27). You are trying to release the tension in the neck and upper back. If you do this correctly, the receiver's head will roll around a bit. Next, using your thumbs, make circles under the shoulders with firm pressure. Keep circling and slide toward the neck along the trapezius muscles (see figure 28). When your thumbs meet in the middle under the neck, lift the thumbs and place the hands on the chest and glide out to the shoulders again. Repeat the thumb circles again. This movement is the most important for neck and shoulder relaxation, as this area is a very common place to store tension.

Upper Back

The receiver is still lying on the floor, facing up. Don't have the person turn over yet. You can deliver an excellent upper back massage in this

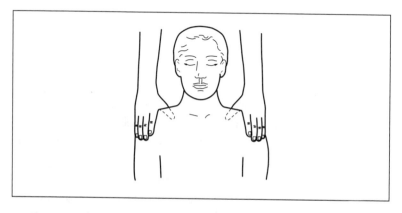

Figure 26. Place your hands on the round part of the shoulders, thumbs underneath, with your fingers pointing down the length of the arms.

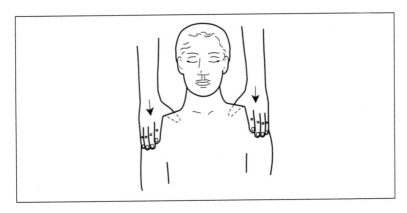

Figure 27. Press each shoulder, one at a time, toward the feet of the receiver.

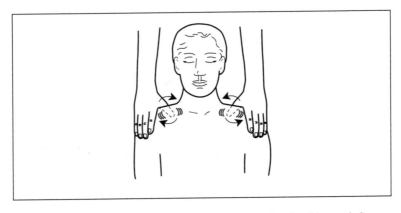

Figure 28. Using your thumbs, make circles under the shoulders with firm pressure. Keep circling and slide toward the neck along the trapezius muscles.

position, using the weight of the receiver to counteract the pressure your hands will deliver. With both hands simultaneously, reach under the receiver's back by sliding the backs of your hand against the floor. Wiggle down, inch-by-inch, with flat hands until you have arrived halfway down the back. Your hands will be on either side of the spine. Cup your hands slightly to deliver pressure from the fingertips and slide your hands slowly up the back toward the neck. When you get to the top, inch your way back down again and repeat the move as many times as you'd like.

Before You Turn the Person Over

You may perform the same movements for arms, hands, legs, and feet that you've already learned in the recliner. Simply kneel or sit facing each limb, oil up, and do your favorite progression of movements!

Full Back

Have the receiver lie on the floor, face down. You may cover him or her with a sheet or blanket. Fold the covering down to the buttocks, exposing the entire back. *Do not sit on the buttocks of the receiver—it puts too much pressure on the lower back.* Instead, take a kneeling position beside the buttocks of the receiver, facing the person's head. Apply a liberal amount of oil or lotion to your hands and then using gliding strokes with open hands to the receiver's back.

The first stroke I want you to try will start at the lower back and travel up to the neck. Begin by placing your open hands flat on the small of the person's back, just above the buttocks. Your fingers should point straight toward the receiver's head (see figure 29). With straight arms, press down into the floor and slowly slide up the back (see figure 30). When you get to the top, separate your hands and glide out to the shoulders. Continue sliding as you pass over the shoulders and down the entire length of the arms until you get to the hands (see figure 31).

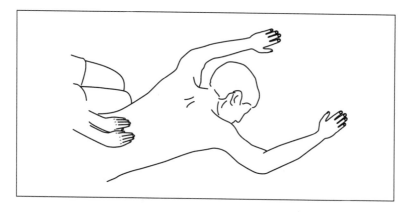

Figure 29. Place your open hands flat on the small of the person's back, just above the buttocks. Your fingers should point straight toward the receiver's head.

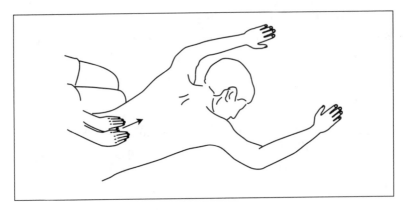

Figure 30. With straight arms, press down into the floor
and slowly slide up the back.

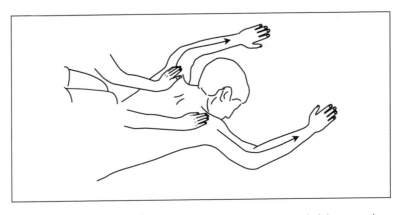

Figure 31. When you get to the top, separate your hands and glide out to the
shoulders. Continue sliding as you pass over the shoulders and down the
entire length of the arms until you get to the hands.

Leave the hands quickly and return to the lower back for another pass.
As you do this move, use your upper body weight to deliver the pressure
to the receiver. Make sure your arms are straight; don't let your elbows
bend. The pressure is delivered when you lean over the receiver's body.

Now try the same pass over the back from the lower back to the
neck, but this time make circles with the upper half of your hands and

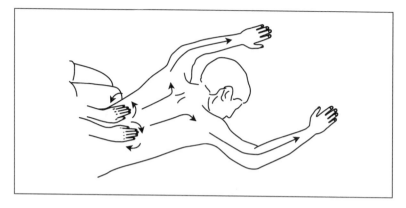

Figure 32. Try the same pass over the back from the lower
back to the neck (as in figure 30), but this time make circles
with the upper half of your hands and fingers.

fingers (see figure 32). When you get to the neck, slide out to the
shoulders and return down the arms as before.

Thumb Sliding

A great move to do on the back is thumb sliding and circling. Place
your hands at the receiver's waist as if you are measuring the person.
Your thumbs will be pointed toward each other on either side of the
spine. Now press the thumbs down into the receiver's body and slide
up the back with even pressure. Remember to use your body weight to
deliver the pressure. When you get to the top, relax the pressure and
slide your entire palms back down the sides of the back and return to
the starting position. After a few passes, repeat this path, but circle
your thumbs up both sides of the spine.

Legs and Feet

The receiver should lie face down, legs spread apart slightly. Roll the
sheet or blanket off one leg to the space between the legs. Apply oil or
lotion to your hands and with gliding motions apply to the entire back
of the leg. You should be in a kneeling position beside the receiver's
knee. You will use the flat palms of your hands to make smooth circles

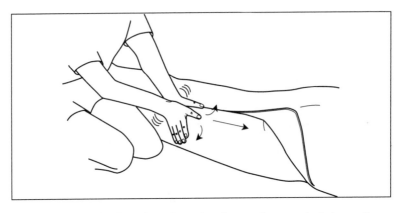

Figure 33. Use the flat palms of your hands to make smooth circles up the back of the thigh from the knee to the buttocks.

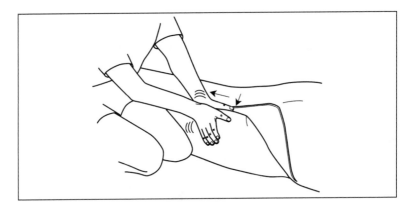

Figure 34. When you get to the buttocks, slide back down slowly as if you're trying to squeeze the thigh between your hands.

up the back of the thigh from the knee to the buttocks (see figure 33). Try to use your body weight to deliver the pressure. I find that it's easier to perform this movement if my hands circle outwardly. When you get to the buttocks, slide back down slowly as if you're trying to squeeze the thigh between your hands (figure 34). Repeat several times.

Now circle your thumbs up the back of the thigh just as you did on the back. Use medium pressure until you feel the hamstring muscle get softer, then you may use deeper pressure. Never apply heavy pressure to the back of the knee, because you can grind the kneecap into the floor.

Hints for Massage at Home

Now that you know the moves, you can create your own routine or pattern to perform a full body massage. A massage session can involve an entire hour or just a few minutes, depending on your daily schedule. Get your practice in, even if you can't carve out time for a long session. Massage is always delightful, even in bits and pieces.

Take It Slowly

Never try to be too ambitious on your first time giving a massage. Your own hands will need to develop muscle stamina in order to do a full body massage. Start out by using this book in stages. Learn the moves one step at a time. For beginners, I recommend massaging for only 15 minutes at a time.

Take Turns

Don't set out to massage each other on the same night. What happens with most couples I've taught is that they get so relaxed receiving a massage that they are often reluctant to get up immediately and give a massage. I suggest that you rotate nights of giving and receiving to avoid hurt feelings.

Communicate

Always let your partner know if the pressure is right. Be supportive and compliment each other when the massage feels good. Avoid being too critical in the beginning. It takes time to develop the movements correctly. Intuition for each other's desires will develop in time.

TWIN FOOT MASSAGES

This is a great way for you and your mate to spend time together, even while watching a movie or your favorite TV show. Lie at opposite ends of the couch with your feet in each others' laps. Use lotion or oil and massage each other's feet.

Aromatherapy

AROMATHERAPY WILL OPEN UP a whole new world for you and everyone in your home. Very simply, aromatherapy is the introduction of smells to effect changes in our bodies. Numerous scientific studies have proved that physiological changes occur by the introduction of aromas though the sense of smell. Specifically, smells affect the olfactory nerve in the nose and cause changes in the brainwaves. We react in a therapeutic way when our noses detect pleasant aromas.

Ancient healers used plant oils for many remedies. In the spa industry, essential oils are used externally to promote relaxation and energy stimulation. Encephalographs have identified which essential oils trigger a reaction in the brainwaves. We can use this information to know which essential oils will produce relaxation and energization.

If you are pregnant or nursing, please consult your doctor before trying these aromatherapy recipes. *Please do not apply essential oils directly to your skin, as the skin is hypersensitive during pregnancy and lactation.*

ESSENTIAL OILS AND EXTRACTS

You are probably familiar with extracts because you've seen them in the grocery store or have used them to bake cookies and sauces. Extracts can be natural or imitation and are generally used for cooking to enhance the flavors of foods. A more pure form of plant extracts is essential oil. You've already been in contact with many essential oils. When you peel an orange, that wonderful fresh orange smell is released into the air because of the tiny capsules of orange essential oil that burst when the skin is removed. When you pluck a rose petal from the stem, a light scent of rose oil can be detected. Essential oils are any oils extracted from plants. True essential oils are extracted through steam distillation and are generally the only recommended essential oils. Essential oils may be used for many different remedies and therapies. I will discuss external use only. For use in the home, I'll identify those essential oils commonly used for relaxing and energizing.

Common Essential Oils and Their Uses

Orange *(Citrus sinensis)* is derived from sweet orange skin. Calming, antigenic, (produces antibodies), and humectant (plumps up dry skin), it is excellent in baths to revive wrinkled skin. Use just a drop or two, because it may irritate sensitive skin. The fragrance of orange is uplifting to most people.

Lavender *(Lavandula agustifolia)* is derived from the flowers and leaves of wild lavender. Calming and soothing to the nervous system, it can help to relieve insomnia, anxiety, headaches, and depression. The word *lavender* comes from the Latin word *lavare,* "to wash." Lavender is widely used for bathing, soothing, and disinfecting. A few drops of lavender added to 1 cup of water can disinfect wounds. Add 20 drops of lavender to your bath water for a soothing bath or add a few drops to your washcloth for a relaxing facial cleansing.

Rosemary *(Rosmarinus officinalis)* is obtained from the stalks, leaves, and flowers of the plant. The fragrance may be very familiar to you. It smells like camphor and is used in many cough drops and cold medicines. It is an antioxidant and may be readily absorbed into the skin. Its properties are stimulating for the mind and memory. A whiff of rosemary in the morning is like a cup of coffee.

Caution: Rosemary should not be used during pregnancy or by individuals with high blood pressure or anyone subject to seizures.

Peppermint *(Mentha piperita)* oil is distilled from the peppermint plant leaves. Peppermint is a familiar scent because it is commonly used in gum, candy, cooking, and even toothpaste. Peppermint oil is an antiseptic, analgesic, and sedative. When used topically, it has cooling properties and is widely used in foot products. Inhaling peppermint can uplift your spirits. Add a few drops to your bath water to cool a fever. Add a few drops to a compress to halt the itch and pain of insect bites.

Eucalyptus *(Eucalyptus globulous)* oil, harvested from eucalyptus trees native to Australia, has a distinctive smell and is used very effectively in cold and sinus remedies. Eucalyptus oil, inhaled or rubbed into the chest, helps clear respiratory and nasal passages. Eucalyptus oil added to a bath will help as an antiseptic.

Lemon *(Citrus limon)* oil, distilled from the peel of lemons, has a fresh scent and helps stimulate the central nervous system. Lemon oil is used in many European countries to detoxify and purify the body. It helps treat oily skin, because of its acidic properties, and is good for dry, brittle nails.

Basil *(Ocimum basilicum)* makes a terrific bath and hair oil. It can help relieve mental stress, depression, and memory loss. Add a few drops to your bath after a stressful or mentally fatiguing day.

Tea Tree *(Melaleuca alternifolia)* is grown in Australia and was widely used for thousands of years by the Aborigines. This lightly fragrant oil is very popular for its antiseptic, nonirritating, soothing qualities. Tea tree oil is frequently used in shampoos and conditioners because it has been said to aid in controlling dry scalp and dandruff. When applied directly to the skin, tea tree helps treat acne, rashes, and fungal infections.

Ylang Ylang *(Cananga odorata)* is my favorite; it has an exotic warm scent. It is widely used in perfumes for its deep fragrance. Ylang ylang can soothe anger and physical pain. It has been known to promote a sense of euphoria, act as a sedative, and treat depression and insomnia. This oil is excellent in baths and as an inhaler and may be applied directly to the skin. It will treat acne and oily skin. The only drawback is that it's very expensive.

Essential Oils at Home

Essential oils may be purchased at health food stores, at retail outlets, or on the Internet. I offer them on my Web site (www.lauradupriest .com). Some oils are relatively inexpensive and some are very costly, due to the nature of extraction. The important thing to remember is that essential oils are in their purest form and are very potent. Use only a drop or two.

Before experimenting with blending different oils, I recommend buying a book that outlines oils and their uses. *Some essential oils can be toxic and should be used with caution.*

For the most part, it is best to inhale essential oils. Simply place a drop in the palm of your hand, rub your hands together, cup your hands over the nose, and inhale. Enjoy the scent slowly as you breathe in deeply.

You may also add essential oils to your bath water or put them on a washcloth for cleansing the face or body. *Remember, just use a drop or two.* (Exception: You may use up to 20 drops of lavender in bath water.)

Making Your Own Massage Oil

A good massage oil should be lightweight, easy to wash off, and should lubricate the skin. I like to blend canola oil with a more exotic oil to make good carrier oil. A carrier oil is used to "carry" essential oils to the skin. Once you have your favorite carrier oil, then you can experiment with adding drops of essential oils to the mix. Other oils to blend with canola oil are sweet almond, grapeseed, sunflower, peanut, olive, and sesame oil. Some of these oils require refrigeration to keep them from going rancid. I recommend that you store your carrier oil in a marked bottle in the refrigerator just to be safe.

> ## HOME SWEET HOME
>
>
>
> *Make your home an oasis with music, candles, and aromatherapy. Your home should be a special place of peace and comfort.*

Skin Irritants

Some essential oils might irritate sensitive skin and should be used with caution, even in bath water. These include citrus oils, cinnamon, peppermint, anise, fennel, and basil.

The Bath

MOST PEOPLE HAVE A bathtub at home, and it's the perfect place to enjoy the spa experience. Soaking and bathing are time-honored rituals. Today we often take quick showers for cleansing only, but with our hectic schedules, we should be kind to ourselves and restore the bathing ritual.

Relaxing in the bath produces instant benefits for the mind and body. Bathing in warm water can soften the skin, relax sore and tired muscles, release tension, calm the nerves, and exfoliate dry skin. Even a ten-minute soak can "slow us down" and help us to enjoy our home and families. The privacy of a bath can help us escape from pressures outside and inside the home as well.

Here are some classic recipes for a myriad of delightful bath treatments. Use them for your own enjoyment, and make the recipes up in decorative jars and tins to give as gifts.

EGYPTIAN-STYLE MILK BATH

For smoothing and softening the skin.

2 TABLESPOONS REGULAR OATMEAL

1 CUP POWDERED MILK

2 TABLESPOONS ALMOND MEAL*

2 TO 3 DROPS OF YOUR FAVORITE ESSENTIAL OIL

*G*rind up regular oatmeal to a fine powder and combine all ingredients in a small bowl. Store in your favorite jar. For a relaxing bath, add 2 tablespoons to bath water and soak for 20 minutes. Afterward, your skin will be remarkably soft and smooth.

*Grind up 10 fresh almonds in a food processor if you can't purchase almond meal.

Modern-Day Milk Bath

*This recipe has the same effect of softening the skin,
but also relieves sore muscles because of the salts.*

1 CUP POWDERED MILK

½ CUP EPSOM SALTS

1 TABLESPOON BAKING SODA

1 TABLESPOON CORNSTARCH

2 TO 3 DROPS OF YOUR FAVORITE ESSENTIAL OIL

$\mathcal{M}$ix all of the ingredients in a bowl and store in your favorite jar. Use 2 tablespoons in a full bath. Soak all of your cares away for 20 minutes.

Bath Salts

Before you learn to how to make bath salts, let's discuss the many uses of bath salts:

+ To soften hard water
+ To soften and tone the skin
+ To relieve tired and sore muscles
+ To help your body recover faster from strenuous work or sports
+ As a great prelude to a body massage to increase your muscles' ability to relax

Making bath salts is easy and fun. You can make up a small batch for immediate use or a larger batch to store for later. For home use I recommend storage in a plastic jar to avoid accidents or breakage around tub and tile surfaces. You may make up bath salts and store them in fancy glass jars to give as gifts.

Aromatherapy Bath Salts

❦

1 CUP EPSOM SALTS OR DEAD SEA SALT
2 TO 3 DROPS OF YOUR FAVORITE ESSENTIAL OIL
1 DROP FOOD COLORING (OPTIONAL)

Stir the salt in a small bowl as you add a drop at a time of the oil and coloring. You will be delighted at how instantly appealing your mix will be. Use 1 to 2 tablespoons in a full bath of water. Soak for as long as you'd like. Towel dry and enjoy how good you feel.

Aromatherapy Bath Fizzies

Effervescent tablets for the bath are a wonderful new addition to the spa market-place. Children, as well as adults, can enjoy a warm bath with aromatherapy fizzies. Making them is so simple, even your children can do it with supervision.

❦

EFFERVESCENT TABLETS (LIKE ALKA SELTZER)
YOUR FAVORITE ESSENTIAL OIL

Place the tablets on a plate. Add only one drop of essential oil to each tablet. Allow 10 minutes for the oil to penetrate the tablets. Store the tablets in a plastic container with a lid or in a decorative bottle or jar. The active ingredient in the tablets is sodium citrate, another form of salt that makes a great bath soak. Add 2 to 3 tablets to a tub of warm water and enjoy.

Recommended oils for bath salts or fizzies: tea tree, eucalyptus, lavender, orange, ylang ylang, myrtle, Peru balsam, and sandalwood.

SWEET DREAMS

Reward your children with a candlelight bath and an aromatherapy massage before bedtime. They will not only love the time you spend with them, they will not fight going to sleep.

Foot Soak Salts

Most experts in the field agree that the best therapy for feet revolves around pepper-mint for its cooling and antiseptic properties. Here's a fragrant foot-soaking recipe to soothe tired, aching feet, which will also treat athlete's foot and fungal problems.

❧

1 cup Epsom salts
2 drops peppermint essential oil
2 drops lavender essential oil
1 drop tea tree essential oil
1 drop green food coloring (optional)

Stir salt in a small bowl while adding oils and coloring a drop at a time to evenly disperse. Store in your favorite jar. Use 1 tablespoon in a small tub and soak your feet for 20 minutes.

Foot-Soaking Fizzies

These are just like the Aromatherapy Bath Fizzies, but peppermint oil is used for the feet.

❧

Effervescent tablets (like Alka Seltzer)
Peppermint essential oil

Place the tablets on a plate. Add only one drop of essential oil to each tablet. Allow 10 minutes for the oil to penetrate the tablets. Store the tablets in a plastic container with a lid or in a decorative bottle or jar. Add one tablet to a foot-soaking tub for a refreshing foot therapy.

Manicures and Hand Treatments

Giving yourself or someone you love a manicure is easy and fun. Most of the time, I recommend a manicure once a week to keep the nails trimmed and cuticles groomed and healthy.

Basic Manicure

Small bowl for soaking

Lotion or hand cream

2 hand towels

Orangewood stick

Cotton

Nail nippers

Nail clippers

Emery board

Cuticle oil, vegetable oil, or margarine

Polish remover

Nail polish (optional)

The best place to give a manicure is sitting at the kitchen table or at a TV table. Fill a small bowl with warm water and lotion (1 tablespoon lotion to 1 cup water), not soap or detergent. (The reason to soak the nails is to soften the cuticles. Soap will do this, but will also dry out your skin.) Place both of the hands in the bowl and soak for at least five minutes. Blot the excess water off with a towel and begin with cuticle grooming.

Take an orangewood stick and wrap a small piece of cotton around the tip to pad it a little. The cuticles simply need to be loosened from the hard bed of the nail; they don't really need to be shoved back. Be gentle and run the padded stick around the rim of the cuticle. This should be fairly easy if you soaked the hands long enough.

Next, trim any hangnails with a nail nipper. (Nippers can be purchased at any drugstore.)

Clip the nails if you want them a lot shorter. Remember to trim the nails straight across, not in a curve. Shaping the nails comes next with an emery board. Work slowly with light pressure until you get to know the amount of pressure your recipient can tolerate.

Now it's time for the relaxing part, the hand and arm massage. First apply a drop of oil to each nail to relieve dryness of the cuticles. A commercial cuticle oil will work, but if you don't have one, just use a drop of whatever oil is in your kitchen, or try a dab of margarine from the fridge. Now apply some hand or body lotion to your hands and begin the hand and arm massage I described earlier in the massage section.

Last, decide if you want to apply polish. Remove the oils from the nail plate by rubbing the nails with polish remover. This will ensure the bonding of the nail polish.

Apply a base coat thinly, then two coats of the colored polish, and finally a top coat. You'll be proud of the first manicure you give!

Homemade Paraffin Treatment for Hands or Feet

1 POUND PARAFFIN WAX

½ CUP SWEET ALMOND OIL

6 DROPS LAVENDER ESSENTIAL OIL

Melt the wax on the stove on low heat. Add the almond oil and essential oil. Remove from the heat and pour the mixture into a plastic container with a lid for later storage. Wait about five minutes until the wax has cooled slightly. Test the temperature with a quick dip of your finger. Apply a thick coating of almond oil or heavy lotion to your hands, then dip your hands into the paraffin bath. Leave the coating on your hands for at least five minutes, then peel off over a trash can. Voila! Instantly your hands will be deeply moisturized, just as with a salon treatment. Place a lid on the container and save for the next time. Each time you use the wax, it will need to be reheated on the stove. Paraffin does not melt in the microwave.

Salon-Style Hand Treatment

If you've ever had a salon-style paraffin treatment, you know how soft your hands feel afterward and what a great prelude it is to a manicure. Here's a wonderful and effective substitute if you don't have access to a paraffin tub at home. You'll need to enjoy at least 15 minutes of downtime.

TWO OVEN MITTS (THE MITTENS YOU WEAR
FOR TAKING HOT THINGS OUT OF THE OVEN)
HEAVY HAND CREAM OR VEGETABLE SHORTENING OR MARGARINE
TWO LARGE PLASTIC BAGS

$\mathcal{D}$ampen the mitts with water in the sink, wring them out so they are just damp, then microwave them for a minute at a time until they are warm, not hot. Smear a good amount of hand cream, margarine, or shortening on your hands. Place hands in plastic bags, and then set them inside the mitts. Sit and relax for at least 10 minutes to give the cream a chance to lubricate your hands in the warm mitts. Remove the mitts and bags, blot off the excess cream or margarine or shortening, and proceed with your manicure.

HAND RESCUE TREATMENT BALM

½ CUP ALMOND OIL
½ CUP HAZELNUT OIL
3 DROPS PEPPERMINT ESSENTIAL OIL
3 DROPS LAVENDER OIL
4 TABLESPOONS BEESWAX

$\mathcal{T}$**he Blend Method:** Combine oils and heat on low for three minutes. In a double boiler, heat beeswax just until melted. Pour oils into a glass or metal bowl while drizzling in beeswax, and whisk together. Let set for one hour. Apply generous amount to hands. Leave on for 10 minutes. Wipe off excess. Will make hands smooth and soft.

The Simpler Method: Combine oils and heat on low for three minutes. Add beeswax and stir until melted. Remove from heat and pour into a plastic jar with lid. Let set for one hour. Apply generous amount to hands. Leave on for 10 minutes. Wipe off excess. Will make hands smooth and soft.

Pedicures and Foot Treatments

YOU CAN GIVE YOURSELF a pedicure treatment, or, even better, get a pedicure from your mate. It's relatively easy and a great indulgence.

HOME PEDICURE

*I find that the best place to have a pedicure is in a recliner, but starting
in the upright position. The feet will be soaked while sitting up, and
then the pedicure can be performed while the receiver is reclining.
I might also add that pedicures are a necessity, because when your
feet are in great shape, life is a lot more tolerable. If your feet are sore
or toenails are too long, even walking can be a chore.*

2 LARGE TOWELS

SMALL PLASTIC TUB FOR SOAKING FEET

(A SQUARE DISHWASHING TUB IS PERFECT)*

FOOT SOAK SALTS (SEE PAGE 199) OR FOOT-SOAKING FIZZIES (SEE PAGE 199)

2 SMALL HAND TOWELS

TOENAIL CLIPPERS

ORANGEWOOD STICK

COTTON BALL

EMERY BOARD

CALLOUS FILE OR PUMICE STONE

MASSAGE OIL OR LOTION

TOE SEPARATORS (IF YOU ARE USING NAIL POLISH)

SPA PEDICURE SET-UP

$\mathcal{P}$lace a large bath towel folded in half on the floor directly in front of the recliner. Fill the soaking tub with very warm water and add 1 tablespoon of your favorite foot-soaking salts or fizzies.

*Many drugstores now sell a foot spa especially for home pedicures; prices will range from $19 to 35 and may feature jets and a heating unit.

Place the tub on the towel in front of the recliner. Have the receiver sit in the recliner and put his or her feet in the footbath. It is best for the receiver to wear a robe or shorts to expose the feet and legs. The giver may gather up the tools and towels while the receiver is soaking. Soaking time can vary by preference, 10 to 20 minutes.

If a recliner is not available, have the receiver sit in any comfortable chair, and set the tub on a large bath towel on the floor at the foot of the chair.

After the foot soak, you'll need to raise the receiver's feet. If you are using a recliner, raise the chair lever to lift the feet out of the footbath and have your second bath towel ready to place under the legs while the chair footrest pops up. The towel will protect the furniture from dripping water. The giver should now get a small stool, ottoman, or chair to sit at the receiver's feet. One hand towel will be used for the giver's lap and the other to dry off the receiver's legs and feet. Once you are in position, follow these basic steps:

1. **Clip Toenails:** Toenails grow at an average rate of $\frac{1}{16}$ to $\frac{1}{8}$ of an inch per month. If the toenails are not trimmed on a regular basis, your feet may become sore from your toenails hitting against the insides of your shoes. Shortening the toenails should be done very carefully with a proper toenail clipper. Unfortunately, most toenail clippers that are sold over the counter have a curved tip. This curved shape can cause you to cut the skin on the sides of the toenails, so I don't recommend this kind of clipper. A professional toenail clipper will have a straight tip. If you can find this kind of tool, take very good care of it, as they are rare.

   When clipping the toenails, always clip them straight across the tip. Avoid rounding and following the shape of the tip of the toe, even though it may be tempting. Curving the nail at the tip can lead to ingrown toenails. The problem will develop slowly over time and can eventually be very painful.

   To clip, hold the foot firmly in one hand, with the fingers securing the toe to be trimmed. If the receiver is jumpy or ticklish, grip the foot more firmly and try again. The clippers are designed to trim the nail only and not any skin. For your first attempt at trimming someone else's toenails, clip small bits until you get the hang of it.

2. **Push Back the Cuticles:** I'm having you do this before you file and smooth the toenails, because this step roughs up the top of the toenails a bit. We want to smooth and file the toenail *after* the cuticle pushing. You will find that the cuticles are very easy to manipulate after the refreshing foot soak. It is necessary to relieve the cuticle skin from the surface of the toenails about once a month. In some cases I've seen over the years, people with very dry, neglected cuticles have ended up with the cuticle growing out with the nails and semipermanently stuck to the nail plate. To keep your nails and toenails in healthy condition, keep the toenails free of the cuticles.

Now, relieving the cuticles should be accomplished with an orange-wood stick that has a tiny bit of cotton wrapped around the tip. This will cushion the sharpness of the stick and prevent "jumpy" feet. The goal here is to loosen the cuticle from the nail plate, but not necessarily shove it way back, which may be painful. Start on one side of the cuticle track, near the tip of the toenail. Trace around the cuticle edge all the way to the other side. You may see fringes of dry skin appear as you do this; that is perfectly normal. The dry skin will be smoothed away in the next step.

After tracing around each toe on the first foot, gently clean under each nail with the cotton tipped end of the orangewood stick. Push the stick outward from the center of the toenail edge to the sides. This will also remove the dead skin from under the nails. Wipe each nail with a towel and proceed to the second foot.

3. **File and Smooth the Toenails:** This is an important step for a good pedicure because it will eliminate rough edges that can scratch you or your partner and can ruin socks and pantyhose. Take an emery board and smooth the rough edges by running the board across the end of the toenail. File in one direction only, to prevent shredding of the nail. Angle your file slightly on top of the nail to properly smooth the top of the edge.

4. **Smooth Calloses:** Use a pumice stone or callous file to gently sand away the hardened skin or callous on the heels, ball of the

foot, or underside of the toes. Work slowly with gentle pressure to avoid sanding normal skin. It will help if you dip the file or stone in water as you work. Keep feeling the area you are trying to smooth with your fingertips to assess how much callous you should reduce. Remember that callous is for protection and should be smoothed but not entirely removed. Taking away too much callous can cause feet to be sore.

5. **Massage the Feet and Legs:** Apply lotion or massage oil to your hands and perform a leg and foot massage, as described in the massage section. Work slowly with firm pressure.

6. **Polish the Toenails:** If polish is desired, remove surface oils by rubbing the toenail surfaces with acetone or polish remover on a cotton ball. A base coat or clear polish is recommended first to keep colored polish from staining the toenails. Before you start, place toe separators or cotton between the toes to keep them from touching each other.

Polishing with color is tricky at first, but you will get the hang of it with practice. The best way to apply polish is to place the brush in the center of the toenail, push the tip back to the cuticle, and then stroke down toward the tip. Apply another stroke to the right of center, and a third stroke to the left of center. For smaller toenails, you can probably cover the nail with one stroke. Apply two coats of colored polish and finish with a clear topcoat. Allow the toenails to dry for at least half an hour before putting on socks or shoes.

Congratulations, you just completed your first pedicure!

MAKE YOUR OWN MARBLE TUB

When giving yourself a pedicure, place some marbles in the bottom of your foot-soaking tub. While you soak, roll your feet around on the marbles for a vigorous massage. Your feet will feel stimulated and refreshed.

Fresh Foot Spray

For a quick pick-me-up after a day on your feet, simply spray on!

½ CUP WATER

½ CUP WITCH HAZEL

10 DROPS PEPPERMINT ESSENTIAL OIL

Combine ingredients in a spray bottle and label. Shake before using.

Foot Powder

*To freshen feet immediately after your morning shower
and to keep feet fresh and cool all day!*

½ CUP BAKING SODA

½ CUP CORNSTARCH

4 DROPS EUCALYPTUS ESSENTIAL OIL

4 DROPS PEPPERMINT ESSENTIAL OIL

Combine baking soda and cornstarch in a small mixing bowl; then add the oils a drop at a time while mixing. Store in a jar or tin. Take a teaspoon of the powder in your hands, then apply to the feet.

Don't wait for a trip to the day spa to begin pampering yourself and those around you! Make your home a place of comfort and relaxation—a retreat from the pressures of stress, work, and chaotic schedules.

Take the time to incorporate what you've just learned into your personal life. By practicing these techniques, you'll engage in a whole new outlook on life—both inside and outside your home.

· 14 ·
Ideas for Children, Babies, and Gifts

"The soul is healed by being with children."
FYODOR DOSTOYEVSKY

"YA MEAN YOU just have to mix that and that to make Chapstick? Then why do ya have to pay for it?"

Kids do say the darndest things, and they do the darndest things sometimes. The information in this chapter offers a twofold benefit: one, it teaches you how to create great spa products in your own kitchen; and two, the experience will provide an opportunity for you to bond with your children. I believe that we should give our kids a chance to be creative in the kitchen. In my kitchen the evolutionary process has gone from cookies and cupcakes to cosmetics.

If you have daughters, they may naturally be eager to learn about recipes for beauty products, but don't count out the curiosity of young boys. My sons, Tony and Johnny, were just past the toddler stage when they began to question why Mom was up to her elbows in experiments on skin masks, cleansers, and scrubs. They saw that I was having fun and they wanted in on the action.

When I started developing my natural beauty recipes for adults, the children naturally ended up underfoot in my kitchen. While I mixed and fussed at the counter, they played with pots and bowls at my feet. That dynamic worked for a while, but they grew up and so did their curiosity. They wanted to help. When they reached ages five and seven, I allowed them to assist in making bath salts. They proved to be terrific at stirring to blend the oils. They were fascinated with the color change that occurred when they added the food coloring. I let them sit up on the counter beside me, stirring and stirring. As they got older, it was their duty to help make batches of products for my salons. As a working mom, I enjoyed the task more while spending time with my boys.

Tony and Johnny are now almost teenagers. Recently, they asked if they could help "invent" something. Their interest in science projects was probably their inspiration. (I explained that using items from the kitchen would probably not fulfill their desire to "blow something up," as in science class.) I was pleased that they expressed an interest and wanted to be in the kitchen with me, so we mapped out a plan.

They needed to come up with a product or an idea. I started them thinking about something that kids needed or kids could use. Once they had an idea, they had to think of the ingredients and test the recipe many times to get it right. Both of them rolled their eyes, as kids often do when their moms talk forever about things they are already aware of. My boys had been through the testing drill for years.

Tony's eyes suddenly lit up, "I want to make hair gel!"

I laughed because he had just received a lecture that morning about the amount of gel he was using to spike up his hair. At age 11, hair was suddenly the focus of his life. (He used an entire tube of professional hair gel each week, an expensive habit.)

"Could you use Jell-O?" he asked.

Then my eyes lit up . . . Gelatin! Maybe it would work! Off we went to the grocery store for unflavored gelatin!

Meanwhile, Johnny was deep in thought. He had no idea what to create. At nine years old, his beauty staples were toothpaste and shampoo. Then I remembered that I'd packed a little jar of Vaseline in his backpack for his chapped lips. Johnny is a fair-skinned redhead, making his skin extra-sensitive. Trying conventional lip balms was tricky because the menthol in most of them usually burned his lips.

"Why not make your own lip balm?" I suggested.

He returned my smile with a scowl, "How the heck do ya do that?"

I didn't have a clue, but I thought it was worth a try. The three of us spent many hours in our kitchen lab over the next few days. Not only did we make hair gel and lip balm, the resulting products performed and tested exceptionally well. Tony's Hair Gel (that's the official name) held his hair as well as, if not better than, the expensive gel. He was surprised that when he got home from school, his hair had not moved. Johnny's Lip Balm (I believe he got the naming technique from his older brother) worked so well that I have added it to my salon aromatherapy line.

My proud little entrepreneurs went off to school, boasting to their buddies about their projects. Both of them sported firm spiky hair and effective lip protection. Upon returning home, they had requests for the products. They were already planning how to spend their money. Like Ben and Jerry's ice cream success, they pictured "Tony and Johnny's" in lights all across America.

They filled a few orders, a bit disappointed at the cost of packaging. Soon, homework and gymnastics practice occupied their lives again. The interesting phenomenon occurred after this experience. They are now more conscious about the price and what's on the label of hair and body products. They have become ingredients detectives.

I wanted to write this chapter to share my boys' experience with other children. Your children will love making natural bath salts and other spa gifts. Chances are, they will do so to give gifts on Mother's Day or for a birthday. Older children may want to try making their own hair gel or lip balm because it's fun and something different to do. (Anything to get them away from the video world.)

The recipes in this chapter are designed for children and babies to use. I have also included recipes that are for all ages, but are easy for children to make. A notation will be made on each recipe to let you know which is age-appropriate. A few of the recipes require cooking and must be supervised. The cooking recipes are not recommended for any child who is inexperienced around a stove. Let the children watch what you are making from across the kitchen at the table. Once the cooking is complete and the recipe has cooled, let them help you put the finishing touches in, such as color and fragrance. They can also help make labels and bottle their projects.

Following the recipes for baby care are ideas for making gifts for all occasions. I receive so many e-mails about the fabulous gifts people make from my recipes. Homemade gifts from the heart bring a smile to the faces of both giver and recipient. Your homemade gifts will look just as dazzling as the spa gifts sold at resorts. The message you send with a gift of relaxation is that you care so much.

For many people, this chapter will bring hours of fun. I wish you great success whether you make items for your own quiet enjoyment or for a loved one. Your creative side will really soar as you dream up ideas for different containers to use for your potions and how to decorate them. Recycled bottles and jars will suddenly become more important to you. I know from personal experience that you'll be more observant when grocery shopping to spot unusual containers that will make the recipes look stunning. To purchase jars, bottles, containers, and even lip balm tubes, log on to my Web site (www.lauradupriest.com).

All of these recipes should be made with adult supervision or help from an adult, and be sure to read each recipe for the appropriate age group.

TONY'S HAIR GEL

Requires cooking, and may not be appropriate for children under eight.

1¼ CUPS WATER

2 ENVELOPES UNFLAVORED GELATIN

1 TABLESPOON PECTIN

1 TEASPOON RUBBING ALCOHOL

1 DROP FOOD COLORING (OPTIONAL)

1 DROP OF YOUR FAVORITE ESSENTIAL OIL (OPTIONAL)

1 EIGHT-OUNCE PLASTIC SQUEEZE BOTTLE WITH A FLIP CAP

*P*our water in saucepan and sprinkle gelatin on top of the water. Let it stand for one minute to soften gelatin. Now turn heat on medium-high. While waiting for it to boil, add the pectin and stir with a whisk. Once the mixture comes to a boil, turn off the heat, but keep stirring for one minute. Let it cool for 10 minutes in a glass measuring cup with a spout. To speed cooling, set the mixture in the refrigerator. Now you may let your little ones finish by adding the alcohol, color, and fragrance. Stir well. The color and fragrance are optional, but the alcohol is necessary to help the gel dry quickly. Make sure you add *just one drop of food coloring*. Little hands want to put in a lot of color, but too much can stain the hair. The essential oil fragrance helps to mask the smell of the alcohol. Try orange, peppermint, lavender, or sandalwood. Pour the gel carefully in the plastic bottle. Affix the lid and shake vigorously. The gel will firm up as it continues to cool. Let your kids shake it occasionally while it sets. Ta da! The gel will be ready to use in about two hours.

Hair gel is great for all ages, but it does get firm and stiff in the hair. I don't recommend it for softer styles that need to be combed. Boys love it because it really holds. To comb it out, simply shower or spray it with a water bottle to soften.

Hint: If your gel is too thick, simply reheat it on low and add a tablespoon of water. Let it cool and re-bottle. If gel is too thin, leave the cap off the bottle for a few days.

GENTLE HAIRSPRAY

This recipe requires cooking; therefore, children eight and under should not participate until the cooling stage is complete.

This hairspray is all natural and helps keep chemicals off children. I realize that most commercial hairsprays are perfectly safe. My children used them with no problems. Still, some children may be sensitive and need help holding hair in place. I never realized that children needed hairspray until mine got involved in school plays, gymnastics, and so on. It seems that young performers, both boys and girls, need starch for their hair. This recipe is a lot like the gel recipe, but diluted. Remember to always have children close their eyes before spraying their hair. The recipe is natural, but it can still sting the eyes.

1 CUP WATER

1 TEASPOON UNFLAVORED GELATIN

JUICE FROM ½ LEMON

1 TABLESPOON KARO SYRUP

1 TEASPOON RUBBING ALCOHOL

2 DROPS OF YOUR FAVORITE ESSENTIAL OIL

1 PLASTIC BOTTLE WITH SPRAY TOP

*P*lace water in a saucepan and sprinkle in gelatin. Let stand for one minute to soften. Add the lemon juice and the Karo syrup and bring to a boil. Remove from heat. Immediately, stir for one minute to blend the ingredients. Let the solution cool for 10 minutes in a glass measuring cup with a spout. Add the alcohol and the fragrance. Pour into a plastic bottle with a spray top. Be sure to label the bottle. This spritz delivers a medium hold. It is safe to use on small children and babies, but do not spray directly on their hair. Instead, spray a little on your fingers and stroke it through the hair for hold.

Note: This spray may lighten hair slightly, so be careful not to use too frequently.

JOHNNY'S LIP BALM

You will be impressed at how simple making lip balm is. The toughest thing is finding the tubes to pour the mixture into. My Web site is a source for tubes, or you

can recycle old Chapstick tubes. Lip balm may also be poured into small plastic
jars or metal tins. This recipe requires cooking; therefore, children under eight
should not participate until the lip balm has completely cooled.

❖

3 TABLESPOONS ALMOND OR VEGETABLE OIL

6 DROPS LAVENDER ESSENTIAL OIL (OPTIONAL)

2 TABLESPOONS BEESWAX PELLETS

CONTAINERS TO HOLD LIP BALM

*H*ave your containers ready. This recipe makes enough to fill six Chapstick tubes or four half-ounce jars. If you have any left over, save it in any small plastic container. It may be reheated in the microwave and poured at a later time.

In a double boiler, heat the oils and wax together. Stir occasionally as the wax pellets melt. As soon as the last pellet starts to disappear, remove the top pan from the boiler. Using a small measuring spoon, carefully fill the tiny tubes, tins, or jars. The mixture will be warm, so be careful. Be sure to fill all containers up to the very top without overflowing. Let your lip balm cool for at least one hour undisturbed. When the containers have completely set, put the lids on. If you used a twist-up Chapstick-type tube, give it a twist and see if your recipe was firm enough. You can always tweak the recipe to suit your needs. If you want a balm that feels moister, use fewer beeswax pellets. If you want the balm to be firmer, use more beeswax pellets. The lavender essential oil is soothing to the lips and very comfortable, even for kids.

Spa Products Children Will Love to Make

BATH SALTS ARE SIMPLE enough to make that even children as young as five years old can accomplish this. Refer to the recipe on page 198. Bath salts can be put in a plain plastic jar with a lid and decorated a number of ways. Let your children's creativity run wild. You can glue dried or plastic flowers to the lid, or attach a label made on a computer. Most children these days can navigate around a computer better than some adults. Glue the label or magazine pictures on the outside of the jar with a glue stick; it works very well. For a finishing touch, tie a pretty ribbon around the neck of the bottle.

You can wrap bath salts in colored cellophane and tie it with a ribbon. It's simple and colorful. Seal the salts in a Ziploc-type bag first so they won't spill when the pretty package is opened up.

Bath salts are sweet gifts for Moms and grandmothers, sisters, and schoolteachers. Dad and grandfathers will love a gift of foot-soaking salts. See recipe on page 199.

Bath Fizzies

The aromatic tablets make bathing fun for children, and your kids will love making them. The task is quick and simple and leaves no mess. The recipe is on page 198. You can package Bath Fizzies the same as Bath Salts. Another idea for a luxurious-looking gift is to package the fizzies in a glass jar with a cork lid. Add a ribbon, label, and flowers. Your children will be proud to say they made this on their own.

Spa Babies

Ahhhhh, the fresh scent of a baby right out of a bath is heavenly. Babies love to be bathed. It relaxes them just as it does adults. Natural recipes for a baby's care may give you peace of mind in knowing how gentle and safe they are. The ingredients in most commercial baby products are many times right under your nose . . . in your kitchen. Baby powders in the marketplace contain talc and corn starch. The great smell you enjoy in baby powder is very mild, but babies don't need the commercial perfume.

Here are three recipes I think you'll enjoy making for your baby or for a friend. Wouldn't it be nice to go to a

Spa Bash

Have a Spa Party for a youngster's birthday. Children can make their own bath salts or hair gel. They will love the creative time in the kitchen and they can take their creation home as a party favor.

friend's baby shower with a gift basket full of homemade natural baby products? The baby gift basket will be the hit at the party and a gift the new mom will always remember.

Note: The essential oils recommended in these recipes are gentle for all skin types, even babies. Perform a skin patch test if you are concerned about allergic reaction. Place a drop of the oil on your fingertip and apply a tiny amount on the back of the baby's upper arm. (This is a safe area that won't end up in the baby's mouth.) If no reaction occurs in 48 hours, the oils are fine for your baby.

Baby Massage Oil

½ CUP CANOLA OIL

½ CUP GRAPESEED OIL

3 DROPS LAVENDER ESSENTIAL OIL

*B*lend and pour in a plastic bottle with a fliptop cap.

Baby Powder

1 CUP CORNSTARCH

½ CUP BAKING SODA

3 DROPS LAVENDER ESSENTIAL OIL

*C*ombine dry ingredients in a sifter. Add oil a drop at a time while sifting. Sift a second time to mix the oil thoroughly. Make a paper funnel and pour into a shaker bottle. A recycled, clean spice jar will do nicely. If you are giving this as a gift, tie a pink or blue ribbon around the neck and make a homemade label.

BABY MILK BATH

1 CUP POWDERED DRY MILK

1 CUP FINELY GROUND OATMEAL (GRIND IN A FOOD PROCESSOR)

3 DROPS LAVENDER ESSENTIAL OIL

3 DROPS SANDALWOOD ESSENTIAL OIL

PLASTIC OR GLASS JAR

Combine all ingredients, stirring very well to blend the oils. Pour into a plastic or glass jar with a lid. Decorate to your heart's content. Add 1 tablespoon of Baby Milk Bath to a tub of warm water. The oatmeal and essential oils will keep baby's skin soft. The powdered milk is a gentle cleanser.

BABY GIFT BASKET

The aforementioned three recipes may be placed in a pink or blue wicker basket. Add some other baby items from the store, such as a washcloth, baby bottles, a plush toy, or teething rings.

SPA SHOWER?

Throw a baby shower for an expectant mother and have the guests make the baby recipes. You can get extra creative with homemade labels for the packaging.

· 15 ·

Salon Secrets
at Home

"By the time you're eighty years old you've learned everything. You only have to remember it." GEORGE BURNS

M Y NATURAL RECIPES for skin and spa care, though created in my kitchen, are really not "top secret," but are commonsense solutions. I'm not the first beauty expert to promote natural recipes, nor do I profess to use them exclusively. I encourage everyone to learn how to take care of their skin with refrigerator and kitchen staples. Practicing natural skin care will lead you to reconsider the high prices at the cosmetics counter. You'll be better equipped to make reasonable purchases of beauty care items.

My crusade in spreading the word about natural ingredients is to inspire you to keep your skin and body looking more radiant and beautiful without the aid of the "secret ingredients" that cosmetics manufacturers boast about. "Secret ingredients" are very rarely a secret.

If you are 35 or older, you may have been a fan of the *Andy Griffith Show,* as I was. I remember a popular episode when Andy was left alone for a week while Aunt Bee went on a trip. Andy's friends were concerned that he wasn't getting any home-cooked meals, so they all invited him over for dinner. Unfortunately, he accepted three invitations for the same night. The episode played out while Andy attended three dinners. All of the hostesses served the same thing: spaghetti. They each claimed to have the best spaghetti sauce because of a secret ingredient. The secret turned out to be oregano. The point is, there is nothing mystical about oregano, but all the ladies who made the dinners were proud of their secret.

In the cosmetics world, once a new chemical or natural ingredient is approved by the FDA, it catapults into the marketplace. Everyone has access to it. The playing field is fairly level, even though manufacturers will try hard to get you to use their "exclusive top secret" formula. I know that after this book, you'll be a smarter shopper and will clearly understand the word *value.*

My recipes for skin and spa care are no more a secret than putting oregano in spaghetti. Many of the recipes work just as well as salon products and services. You may never wish to replace your salon entirely with "at home" service. I hope you don't, because there is nothing quite like having someone else give you a facial or a massage. Visiting a salon from time to time will keep your look current and fresh. You can also learn a lot about how to do your own services at home by watching the professionals. I just hope you realize that what goes on in a salon is nothing mysterious or magical. If you're the type of person who enjoys spoiling yourself at home occasionally, this book provides the "how-to's." Saving money is also a plus. By giving you the power of knowledge, I hope to see a lot more naturally beautiful and happy women out there.

Redesign Yourself

IF I INSPIRED YOU to give yourself a complete or partial makeover, then I accomplished my goal. After so many years of redesigning women, I wanted to take it a step further and help inspire women everywhere, even outside of my salon, to focus on natural beauty. Women need and want to look beautiful. It starts when we are very young, wanting to look nice on the first day of school. It continues throughout our lives with proms, dates, weddings, and everyday life. I want to inspire people to keep up the effort to look great every day. Start with just a few new ideas and begin implementing them a step at a time. Perhaps you are already gathering ideas from magazines and maybe you even put together a "look book." Now, when you shop for clothing, you'll have a better plan for building your wardrobe. Keep adding a new habit each week or month. If you use my shopping tips, staying current with the world of fashion will be a lot easier and more enjoyable.

SMART PRODUCT SHOPPING

Set yourself apart from the rest of the shopping public by being smarter about beauty product spending. Learn to spot the "Snake Oil" and pass on buying it. Find out all you can about a salon or cosmetic product before you rush out to purchase it. Don't forget, the Fountain of Youth was a myth. Creams, lotions, and potions that promise to deliver the Fountain of Youth may have a lot of mythology behind them as well. Your common sense is your best guide to sorting through the hype. Remember that the cosmetics industry spends billions of dollars each year to sell you the myth. You can make the choice of spending lots of money or spending your dollars wisely. Saving money has its own merit. Feeling good about what you purchase will give you a better attitude, and attitude creates outer beauty.

Beauty from the Inside Out

THE MOST IMPORTANT CHAPTER in this book is about the beauty we all have inside ourselves. Experiencing joy in your life will undoubtedly be your best beauty secret. Your inner peace will produce the longest-lasting radiance. When you are happy and content, you will seldom need much makeup at all. Be the kind of person who inspires others with your positive attitude and inner confidence. Once you've mastered the ability to keep your inner beauty constant, you will surely turn heads. If you ever wake up and doubt your image in the mirror, go back and read chapter 5, "Inner Beauty." Always start from the inside out. Looking good will be easier if you beautify your inner self, first and foremost.

My Natural Recipes

THE GREATEST SECRET I'VE tucked away in my natural recipes is the idea of doing something by yourself, for yourself. That's it, in a nutshell. With very little effort, time, or money, you can always indulge yourself with a little pampering. The results will certainly be physically beneficial, but your sense of accomplishment will be greater. Giving yourself a facial or a spa treatment in the privacy of your own home whenever you want is a wonderful joy and freedom. Your time-out for relaxing is an important step toward taking care of your body and soul. If you've never done it before, try to introduce one recipe at a time. Eventually, you may make a habit out of a complete facial once a week. The difference in your skin will be noticeable. The difference in your attitude after taking time for yourself will be a welcome change. Vow that you will no longer neglect yourself!

Spa-ing Partners

WHEN I READ THE e-mails I receive from couples and families about my spa-at-home recipes, I feel fortunate to have helped create a bond between members of a household. The time we spend with our families and loved ones is the most important time we have. When you give your grandmother a pedicure or your husband an aromatherapy massage, your inner beauty thrives because of the service you give to others. Many moms have shared my spa-at-home secrets with teenagers and used my techniques to massage their babies. Life at home will never be the same after you begin to introduce the spa atmosphere. I still honor my pre-teen boys for accomplishments with a massage. They rush to get their chores done if they've been promised an aromatherapy back rub at bedtime. Soothing the chaos in your home is easy with a little knowledge and motivation. Make sure you try the spa techniques on family members so you'll be treated to some spa services as well. Spoil your mate with my techniques and you'll soon have a "spa-ing" partner for life.

You Can Be an Expert

WHEN IT COMES TO your hair and makeup, you can and should be an expert. I never underestimate the knowledge a client has about her own hair and face. You know yourself better than anybody. My ideas about hair and makeup stem from many years of working on hundreds of people in a salon. I learned the secrets from people just like you. From now on, think of yourself as an expert. Consider that I just gave you a master's degree in makeup and hairstyling. You can do it just as artfully as your local salon professional can, you just didn't know all the techniques before now. Trust yourself and keep practicing. You deserve to look beautiful every day, not just the day you leave the salon.

GO TO A SALON OR DO IT YOURSELF

When I first started this project, I was criticized by other salon professionals for cutting myself out of a lot of business. Won't people learn your tricks and not go to the salon? I believe in sharing knowledge. Knowledge is not to be hoarded, but passed on. I didn't develop every single technique I am sharing. I've learned so many things from others who were willing to teach me. There will always be people who never want to do things on their own. Salons will never lack for business. Many services should not be attempted by people at home. I believe this book will send a lot of business to salons, as people become more hungry for relaxation and beautification.

A Change for the Better

IF I'VE CONVINCED YOU to make yourself over, you'll be amazed at the positive benefits of change. It will make you feel fresh, adventuresome, and alive. Change keeps things exciting, and, in many ways, makes us feel young. Keep in mind the analogy of rearranging a room when you think about a makeover. When we move the furniture around in our house, it creates new excitement and a break in our routine. The same thing is true for ourselves. Push toward change every once in a while. You'll reap the benefits.

Better, Faster

TIME DOESN'T HAVE TO be the enemy when it comes to beauty. We can find the time to do things we really want to do. I don't know any woman who doesn't want to be more beautiful. I hope my secrets to looking beautiful will inspire you to let your natural beauty shine. Never think that you have to neglect yourself just because you are busy. You are more important than your schedule. You can make the schedule and pace yourself accordingly. All you need to do is reorganize and create new beauty habits, one step at a time. Time will continue to march on as you look in the mirror, day after day. You can choose to march along with it and feel comfortable that you look your best, despite your age.

The "Natural Beauty" in the Mirror

I WANT YOU TO always admire the beautiful person you see in the mirror. Your mirror is your friend. Never compare yourself to the sea of glamorous faces around you. Your goal should be to strive for the natural "you" and what you want to look like. Start with the beautiful attributes you know you already have and go from there. Natural beauty is easy to achieve if you begin with a little self-admiration. Adding some simple, basic beauty secrets, one step at a time, will give you a new outlook on life. You'll see a difference in the way you look and will feel so much better about yourself.

I hope this book has given you the knowledge and power to feel more in control of how you present yourself. The world of beauty and glamour is easy to enter if you want to. Glamour isn't just for "born lucky" women. Include yourself in the pool of beautiful women. The keys to beauty are not locked up in expensive creams and jars. The keys are sitting right before you and you can use them anytime that you want.

Never walk down the street feeling left out or jealous of other women you feel are more beautiful than you. Learn to admire other beautiful women and learn from them. Make a pledge to enjoy looking and feeling more beautiful. Your own natural beauty will become more apparent to you every day for the rest of your life.

In my continued quest to educate women and help them enjoy natural beauty, I invite your questions and comments. My Web site is www.lauradupriest.com.

Index

230 · *Index*